HAPPY
HEALTHY
FIT

Transform Your Life in 90-Days with
The figure*FIT!* Lifestyle Program.

LIZ NIERZWICKI

Published by Best Seller Publishing®, Pasadena, CA

Best Seller Publishing® is a registered trademark

Printed in the United States of America.

ISBN-13:978-1522871514
ISBN-10:1522871519

This publication is designed to provide accurate and authoritative information with regard to the subject matter covered. It is sold with the understanding that the publisher is not engaged in rendering legal, accounting, or other professional advice. If legal advice or other expert assistance is required, the services of a competent professional should be sought. The opinions expressed by the authors in this book are not endorsed by Best Seller Publishing® and are the sole responsibility of the author rendering the opinion.

Most Best Seller Publishing® titles are available at special quantity discounts for bulk purchases for sales promotions, premiums, fundraising, and educational use. Special versions or book excerpts can also be created to fit specific needs.

For more information, please write:

Best Seller Publishing®

1346 Walnut Street, #205

Pasadena, CA 91106

or call 1(626) 765 9750

Toll Free: 1(844) 850-3500

Visit us online at: www.BestSellerPublishing.org

TABLE OF CONTENTS

DISCLAIMER

The ideas, opinions, and concepts expressed in this book are intended to be used for educational purposes only. This book is sold with the understanding that author and publisher are not rendering medical advice of any kind, nor is this book intended to replace medical advice, nor to diagnose, prescribe or treat any disease, condition, illness or injury. It is imperative that before beginning any diet or exercise program, including any aspect of the figureFIT! Lifestyle Program, you receive full medical clearance from a licensed physician. Author and publisher claim no responsibility to any person or entity for any liability, loss, or damage caused or alleged to be caused directly or indirectly as a result of the use, application or interpretation of the material in this book.

FOREWORD

You're probably reading this because at some point in your life, you've decided that you need to make a change. You don't feel well, are tired, but the traditional medical system may have let you down, or not been able to help despite costly and time-consuming tests and treatments. Or perhaps you'd rather not take medications that you're not comfortable with. In her book, Liz Nierzwicki helps you understand and implement the changes to allow you to take control, and be in charge of your life, using the latest advances in the science of fitness and dietetics.

There is a paradigm shift in medicine happening in medicine today. We are realizing that the humanistic aspect of medical care has often been missing, yet is critical for the total health of the patient. Health and well being isn't just about having good numbers like blood pressure or cholesterol. It's about having the full spectrum of emotional, spiritual, and physical health that makes one whole. From our population health studies, understand this regarding what influences the health outcomes of patients:

- Our genetics – 20%

- Socioeconomic environment -20%

- Medical care, access and quality—an amazingly low 10%

- *Patient behavior—50%*

Unfortunately, although the best medical doctors may be great at making the diagnosis and recommending the best treatments available, we are still dependent on the patients to follow through once they leave our office. Liz delivers fascinating insights into why some succeed while others may fail even though they know what they must do to improve…but can't. And for physicians like me, that is the secret sauce in getting people healthy, and happy—not their medications, but changing behaviors.

Define what it means to be healthy. Some say health is wealth. Medical bills account for the vast majority of bankruptcies today. By staying healthy, we can avoid those catastrophes especially as we age. Others say being healthy means not getting sick or being sick.

But I say also, it means *not feeling sick*. So often, I see people in my office that "don't feel well", convinced that they have an illness, yet we cannot find any evident medical problem. There's a different definition of health, and that is the "Sense of Well-Being". I believe that's what Liz is getting at in this book. We can have a patient with cancer, or someone with a chronic illness that is not curable such as diabetes, but they actually feel healthier than someone without any disease. Why?

By this time you may realize that what it means to be healthy is to feel good—physically, emotionally, and spiritually…regardless of one's prognosis or underlying genetics or social condition. Liz talks in her book about the importance of loving oneself. Not in a self-serving superficial way, but rather a deep understanding of one's own vulnerabilities and faults, and a willingness to address them. I believe as a Catholic that we are given unconditional love, and we need to love ourselves before we can truly unconditionally love others.

It will take work and it will take time, but it will be a labor of love. And you can start that process now.

PREFACE

Hello, my new friend. I am super excited that you picked up this book and that you are interested in learning my philosophy and tools for a healthy digestive system, FIT body, and happy mind.

My name is Elizabeth Nierzwicki (Liz). I want nothing more than to help you figure out how to become healthy, FIT, and so abundantly happy with your life that you turn into a lighthouse for others.

I know beyond a shadow of a doubt that the tools in this book work. Not only do they work, but they also create massive transformation internally and externally. I am proof that this lifestyle yields substantial results. I am now more fit, stronger, and happier than I have ever been in my whole life. I am psyched to help you fall completely in love with yourself and your body, which I call your holy home.

For as long as I can remember, I have been a seeker of peace. When I was in my early 20s, I used to spend countless hours reading spiritual books, creating artwork, dancing, and sometimes just sitting and listening to the sounds of my surroundings. Even before that, when I was a little girl, I would spend hours upon hours outdoors. I would ride my bike, play in the woods behind my house, and make mud pies, which I offered to the birds (something fascinated me about the mud). I would also make forts and admire nature while living in my little corner of the world. Little did I know that this was a deeply relaxing and spiritual practice all on its own.

I was the youngest of three siblings. My sister is five years older than me, and my brother is three years older. Looking back on my childhood and having learned child psychology, I have come to understand why my sister did not like me very much when we were growing up. Because when I arrived, everything in the family went to pieces.

My parents split up due to an affair, and it was no longer just her and our brother (her best friend). She became a leader and babysitter fast when my mom needed her. Divorce is difficult for kids, and I think that our parent's divorce was hardest for my sister because she was only five years old and loved her daddy. I, on the other hand, did not know it any other way than how it was – the four of us.

My sister and brother picked on me a lot and excluded me from playing with them and their friends, so I would go off and find my own things to do.

Once, my brother's friends told me that I could not sled on their hill, so I went and found my own, not realizing that it had a 10-foot drop off at the end of it. Yeah, that mishap left me with fractured lower vertebrae, and I was unable to get up and walk. In the moment, I thought I was paralyzed. My brother was a true champion that day and pushed me in my sled all the way up a hill to a friend's house where they called my mom and an ambulance.

My recovery took weeks, and the one thing I remember is the physician telling me that I needed to tighten my core before I did any movement. To this day, I teach the same principle to all of my clients.

Now, as an adult, I can look back at the experiences from my younger years and see how they all brought me to where I am today. I have realized the little things that added up to make me who I am: why I opened a yoga studio (called Solace), what makes me comfortable or uncomfortable, why I like to be alone, and why I have struggled in romantic relationships. Most of all, I have come to learn why I have always been a soul seeker and a seeker of internal solace.

Solace [sol-is]   (*not* soul-less)

Noun, also called solacement

1. Comfort in sorrow, misfortune, or trouble; alleviation of distress or discomfort.

2. Something that gives comfort, consolation, or relief.
   Verb (used with object), solaced, solacing.

3. To comfort, console, or cheer (a person, oneself, the heart, etc.).

4. To alleviate or relieve (sorrow, distress, etc.).

In 2010, I founded Solace Yoga Studio. Little did I realize at the time that I would become a healer and someone who helps people rediscover happiness within themselves. This was the beginning of my journey of understanding who I am and what my true purpose is on this planet. And now I write this book to help you do the same. Opening a yoga studio was not something that I had always dreamed about. It evolved from my natural likes, dislikes, needs, and one of my life goals: becoming an entrepreneur.

To me, a bouquet of love surrounded the word solace. I don't remember when I first heard or read the word, but I found it to be beautiful. The word alone made me feel good, and I thought it was the perfect fit for a yoga studio since it means peace, and yoga was the ultimate stress relief to me.

Unfortunately for me at the time, I wasn't very peaceful internally. Too many things were happening at the same time. I was running a new business and teaching 18 classes per week as a single mother. I loved what I was doing, and my business was like a second child, but I was burning out.

Then in 2012, everything as I knew it changed. That year, my son's father asked me if I would be open to letting our son come and live with him (six and a half hours away), because he wanted to have some influence in our son's life. My son was 10 years old at this time, and he had lived with me up until now.

Instantly it felt like a punch in the gut. *"Why had I never thought that this question was going to come about? Of course, he was going to ask this at some point,"* I thought. I knew in my heart that the decision was already made. Although not a single ounce of me wanted this to happen, I knew it was something that needed to happen for the sake of my son's well-rounded upbringing.

I told my son's father that I would think about it. I knew that I couldn't say, *"Heck no, I won't consider this"* because I knew that my son needed to spend time with his father. I didn't have a father in my life, and I knew that I had missed out on so much because of this. I also knew that I had struggled in relationships because of this lack of fatherly love in my life. A mother who has to pull both mom and dad duties can give a child only so much. There will always be an imbalance on the side of the one who is not in the home. I knew that my son needed a father's influence just as much as he needed mine. He was getting to the age where being around his father would be of utmost importance.

I discussed it with my son, and he said that he wanted to give it a try. The decision was made, and for the next three months, I couldn't look at him without crying. I have been through some major challenges. Being a single mom is tough. Opening a small business is tough. Letting go of the person you love more than anything because it is good for them – that was the most difficult thing I had ever done.

The summer of that year, I spent every last moment I could with my son. I wanted to prepare him for a new life with his father. I also wanted to ensure that he knew that I would always be there for him and that he could come back at any time.

Once he left, I dove into my work at the studio and created Solace Yoga School to begin training and graduating new yoga teachers.

I also dove into a relationship with a man who was very wrong for me on many levels. He was eight years younger than me, and he was from Serbia, so both the differences in age and language went against us. In the back of my mind, I knew that I attached myself to him because my son was now gone (more on this type of behavior later), and he helped filling this void. However, I soon realized that nothing could fill that void except meditation, prayer, and loving myself, so I set out on a journey to do just that.

I loved my business and creating new things, so developing the curriculum for the school was a great adventure for me, and it also gave me something to focus on. In addition, I loved my workouts and how great they made me feel both physically and mentally. Once I opened the yoga studio, I decided to become a personal trainer. I had been training friends and family since 2000, so I figured I should make my training official.

Then I learned about the body's energy systems and how we can get a faster metabolism (among other things) by training them in a specific way. After I turned 33, I noticed that my metabolism had slowed down significantly, so I wanted to use the science for my benefit. I continued my education around this topic and then created workouts at my studio called Body Sculpt (which are now called figureFIT!) to put this science into play. These classes were named Body Sculpt (not yoga classes) because I did not want people to come to the studio expecting a yoga class and then surprise them with lunges and weights and a killer core workout only to have them never come back again because they were expecting a gentle yoga class.

The Body Sculpt workouts started to change my body. I began to have more energy than ever before. I lost weight, and it got to a point where I no longer needed to worry about the foods I ate. I ate normal meals; I had breakfast, lunch, dinner, and if I needed a snack, I would have one. I focused on building my meals around protein but didn't put too much concern into staying away from carbohydrates or fats. I became leaner than I had ever been before, and it was only due to the workouts because that was the only thing that I changed. I was *not* doing cardio training. I was training my body's energy systems.

Once the yoga school was certified by the yoga alliance (yeah, I started a school!), I set out to launch the inaugural yoga teacher training class of 2013. Then I fell in love with training the yogic path. There is a common phrase that says, "To teach is to learn," and that proved to be the case for me. I dove into teaching and loved what this path had to offer. I started to learn more about life, my attachments, mental patterns, and kleshas. Kleshas, a Sanskrit word, are the causes of our suffering. They are "afflictions" that distort our mind and our perceptions, and they affect how we think, act, and feel. I started to unravel the layers that had been built in my mind about life and my body over the years.

Throughout this book, I am going to share stories with you about clients, friends, family, and myself. I hope that you will learn from the life lessons of others so that you can make informed decisions about your life and not fall into the same traps. I am also going to share with you what I have learned over my lifetime of studying the nutrition science, psychology, and the path of yoga.

Most of all, my purpose for writing this book is to share with you what I have come to know and understand. I have learned that we are given the gift of life, and we are given a *holy home* for the soul because our soul is on a mission. I want to help you be as healthy and fit as you can be and find your ultimate purpose in life. It is our obligation to take care of our body so that we can fulfill our duties while we are here. I will show you how to do it with the figureFIT! tools. The tools are necessary for your happiness. When we are not happy, everything else seems like a problem. It's time to take your power into your own hands and implement the tools that will help you develop your body and mind, and create a life you love.

My hope for you is that you begin to know that your body is your holy temple and that you will start to see yourself as extremely valuable and important for the entire planet. Not a single one of us is a mistake. Even though I was an accident for my parents, I know my worth (although it took the practice of self-love to feel this way). The Universe had a plan for me long before I was here. You are the same. When you know your worth and value, and you take care of your body, mind, and spirit, you will have a healthy and happy life beyond your wildest dreams.

Having a healthy mind and body and a happy heart is done when you build a lifestyle that is sustainable for you based on the science of what works. All you have to do is walk the path set forth in this book. You will not have to kill yourself in the gym or on a certain diet to fix yourself. When you understand the science, you can apply the tools, and they will work for you even if you believe that you have "bad genes."

Your body is a gift. We have all heard it called our temple. I hope that you will begin to embrace this concept not just conceptually but with every cell of your body. Begin to love yourself and everything that has gotten you to this point where you are reading this book. The concept is to treat your body like the holy home it is, in need of your love and respect. Live a life that honors your vessel and, therefore, your soul.

When you have a healthy body, you can fulfill your function on this planet. When you do not value your holy home, you will get sick. Then you will have to focus on healing, and that holds you back and gets in the way of your true purpose. I believe we all have a calling, and it's closer to your understanding than you think. It's only when you tap into your self ... through self-care, self-love and meditation that you will understand what that calling is.

This book breaks down what I teach my members of the figureFIT! Lifestyle Program and incorporates everything that is coming mainstream for the health conscious. I will cover where all disease begins, the psychology of change, proper nutrition, the science of meditation, mindset training, yoga, energy system training, weightlifting, high-intensity interval training, and much more.

The time has come to ditch the diet and the all-or-nothing mentality and approach to health. Instead, we should return to what is real and what promotes true health and longevity. And that is simply treating your body (on a daily basis) as the holy home it is. Live a life that supports health and not destruction. That means feeding it the right fuel and training it properly.

Happiness and peace are our birthrights. Now that I'm older, I am very clear that I must dismiss anything that takes me out of my center. I meditate daily for peace of mind and to connect with my spirit. I maintain around 15 percent body fat because I move my body every day. I eat real foods and at the right times. I rarely get sick. When you learn what true health is all about for you, you will become fit, healthy, and happy. That is my promise to you, and I can't wait to hear how this program changes your life.

Being healthy and fit should be cheap and easy and not require drastic measures. We are meant to be well, and I have learned that when we pay attention to our mind, intuition, and body's signals, it's quite easy and natural to be healthy and fit.

I am very aware of the dieting pitfall of cutting calories and the rebounding binge that usually happens to make yourself feel less deprived. Diets don't work because you are not changing the mindset and beliefs behind the behaviors. To fully be who you want to be, you must make it a daily effort; you must make it a lifestyle.

Life is a series of events that help you decide who and what you want to be and what you do and don't want in your life. Your thoughts can be simply programmed habits. Change the thoughts, the stories you tell yourself, and watch your life bloom. Have compassion towards yourself as you are learning and going through these daily life experiences. Allow yourself to be imperfect and know that becoming who you want to be is a series of choices.

I will not sugarcoat this; you will have to look in the mirror and face the fact that your life is your creation. If you do not like where you are, or you want a different reality, you will have to put in the work to change yourself. The beauty is that it's all a simple choice. Life is always up to you. We often make it harder than it needs to be. I am here to help you, so know that you do not have to be stuck in a place that doesn't serve you. It's a choice to live and make decisions from your personal place of power.

I now realize that this is more than a book. It is a centerpiece of a fit family of people connected by the Internet. The people on the figureFIT! Lifestyle Program are all committed to living a healthy life, changing old patterns, and empowering themselves to live the life they want in a healthy body. In all honesty, the figureFIT! Program is about growth. It's about breaking down old habits that keep us stuck and creating new habits that support health and wellness in the body and spirit.

The power is in the doing, so I encourage you to sign up for the monthly online figureFIT! Lifestyle Program at figurefitlife.com so that you can fully embody the principles of this lifestyle.

One of the most important parts of any transformation is finding people who understand what you are going through or have been through it. Your new fitness family is here in the figureFIT! community. When you lock arms with people on the same mission, you have people to be accountable to and to support, and that in turn helps you to be accountable to yourself. In the private figureFIT! community, you will have me, my assistants, other trainers and coaches, as well as all of the members on the program. We are all there to support *you* and help you grow into who you envision yourself to be – beautiful, vibrant, healthy, and living your dreams!

Real peace comes from being connected and knowing that others are going through the same experiences as you are. I have found that when I am ashamed of where I am in life and then share my story with someone I trust, I am met with love. I realize that I never had anything to fear. Beyond that, my sharing always gives others encouragement to make a change in their life. So I encourage you to join the monthly program, share your story with us, and never be ashamed of where you are or what you're going through. It will allow you to connect with others who are all in a similar situation and can relate to you in a way no book or trainer ever could. When you put into practice what you are learning, you will see changes beyond your wildest dreams.

The figureFIT! Lifestyle Program is a way of life that is attainable for everyone, not just those who are fit and healthy already. It's time to jump in. But know that you will be caught with so much support, love, and guidance that you have no choice but to succeed.

I have learned that my mission on this planet is to help people find their inner peace and cultivate balance between life, self-love, health, and spirituality so that they know *who* they are and can live a life of true passion and purpose. I hope that this book will serve you and help you to become the best version of *you*.

My goal is that this book will give you new insight into the human body. I hope that you will gain practical knowledge that you can apply to your life that will help you *and* your family. I want you to take the driver's seat of your life. I will explain the full holistic approach to having (and loving) your holy home (body).

In this book, you will learn about the following:

- Proper nutrition, the gut microbiome, etc.

- How to train the body for what you are looking to do: lose weight, gain muscle, have a better butt, you name it

- The brain and how to manage the monkey-mind

- Yoga, meditation, and managing your stress levels

The busiest and most successful people I know are not the ones who complain about not having enough time for taking care of themselves. They have made themselves a priority because they know that to be successful means having a healthy body.

We are all in the same boat, and it's what you decide to do on a daily basis that matters. We all have the same amount of time in the day. What you choose to focus on is up to you. Know that the law of attraction is real and that you will get what you focus on. Change is not an instantaneous thing. It happens in the process – in the daily life that you live. Then, one day, you will realize you have the body you wanted, you are living the life you dreamed, and most importantly, you're happy and healthy. What is more important than that?

Join the online figure*FIT!* Lifestyle Program.

I used to cry in my closet because I was "too fat" for my clothes. I killed calories in the gym after binging the night before. I've scolded myself time and time again over my body, but none of that ever worked.

It wasn't until I started seeking help from people who had the body, health, and life I wanted that my life began to change. I dove into books, seminars, and classes to help me learn how to better myself. I hired life, fitness, and nutrition coaches. Some were good, and some were great while others didn't seem to give me a second glance or care about my goals. Eventually, I started learning how to love myself through proper care such as positive thinking, eating the foods that were right for me (listening to my body's signals), and working out the right way.

After years on this journey, I realized I needed to create my own program to help clients. I wanted to create a program that fully integrated fitness, digestive health, healing, and a healthy mindset. I created exactly what I would have wanted help with when I was hiring my coaches. Now here it is *for you*!

With this book *and* my online program, you receive the tools you need to create a solid foundation for a happy mind, a healthy gut, and a strong, sexy body. When you head over to figurefitlife.com and join the online figureFIT! Lifestyle Program, you will receive all the tools you need to make major changes in your life. You will also have direct access to me on a daily basis via the private group page on Facebook.

Change does *not* happen in your comfort zone, so it's time to commit to you, your goals, and your health and start taking steps daily for your happiness and health.

Here is what you receive:

- Three figureFIT! Metabolic Conditioning Workouts per month
- Weightlifting Workouts
- A Monthly Fitness Calendar
- Yoga Videos
- Audio Meditations (self-awareness is key!)
- The figureFIT! Nutrition Guide with Food Lists
- Paleo Recipes
- Private group support page for daily check-ins and support
- Motivating Group Coaching Calls

Self-Love is Where It's At

During our life we go through things that challenge us and rock us to our core. Sometimes we think we are alone in our journey and struggles but then (like magic) the universe delivers us something like this program. You're naturally attracted to people and things that will help you and all of a sudden you end up sharing space with people who are there to help you, support you, and love you while you're beginning to love yourself.

If you're ready to elevate your entire life, body and health, join us at figurefitlife.com and sign up for the monthly online coaching program: the figureFIT! Lifestyle Program. If you want one-on-one help, I do that too and with that you also get access to the monthly online program and your new tribe!

I can't wait to meet you!

INTRODUCTION
You Are More

"God's will for you is perfect happiness."

– ACIM

"I am not a body. I am free as God created me."

– ACIM

Are you happy? Perfect happiness is our goal. We are all entitled to it simply by being alive. Over my years on this planet, I have found that many people are not happy. Nor are they at peace with the world, themselves, their job, their body, and so on. I too spent many years seeking peace.

The cornerstone of the ego's thought system is that you are guilty, powerless, not needed, abandoned, and more. The cornerstone of the spirit, on the other hand, is that you are pure love and entitled to perfect happiness.

Through my studies of nutritional science, psychology, and Eastern yoga philosophy, I have learned a great deal about how to end suffering. You can end the suffering of the body by eating foods that help you rather than harm you. You can heal your mind by understanding how the mind works, letting go of attachments, and meditating. You can heal your heart and become happy by putting into place the tools that will get you there.

In the first few chapters of this book, we will walk through a couple of philosophical ideas together. Then we will move on to the tools and ideas that will help you have a happy, healthy, and FIT life.

Who are you? What do you think this life is all about? Do you believe that we are meant to be happy? Do you feel like life is nothing but a big struggle? These are all extremely important topics, and your beliefs about each question will ultimately determine the outcome of your life.

If you feel that you are destined for greatness and believe that the Universe (or God) has a miraculous plan for you, then I would say you are on the right track. If you think your life is worthless and pointless and that it will always be a struggle, then we have some work to do. If you do not like the word God, insert universal spirit or any description that will connect you to the understanding of a higher power.

I'd like to break down the quotes I started this chapter with: "I am not a body. I am free as God created me." The first part is "I am not a body." This phrase has become one of my favorite things to say to people, especially when they say something to me about their or my body. It took 36 years for this message to sink in for me. Unless you get this message ingrained in your life's philosophy, you are bound for disappointment. You will seek out people based on how they look, and they will do the same to you.

I am not a body; I have a body. If we think we are our body and don't realize we are more than that, we will inevitably become sad or very unhappy as we get older and our body starts to break down, our skin begins sagging, we get wrinkles, and so on.

We live in a society that values the physical – good looks, new cars, the hottest handbag, the cutest boyfriend or girlfriend, etc. These values get deeply ingrained in us through many different mediums. It's not until we get older that we realize none of this gives us true happiness. This idea that our happiness is "out there" has done nothing but teach us to value the valueless.

Think about a time when you are checking out in the grocery store, or you are in the middle of an exchange of some sort, and you have overlooked the person right in front of you. Perhaps you didn't even look at them in the eye, or you simply did not engage in conversation with them because you were "just trying to get your to-do list done?" You are physically there interacting with another person, but are you mentally there? Do you see the beautiful gift of life standing in front of you? Why do we do this? Why not be fully where you are when you are there? Sometimes, we do not see others because we are looking over their shoulder for the next best thing, or we are preoccupied with our problems, on our phone, or talking to someone else. It is sad, and life does not need to be this way, nor should it be this way. Every living being is worthy of more than that, and we need to begin to value the valuable.

You, my friend, are valuable, and so are your children, your friends, your parents, the strangers around you, the dog, the cat, and so on. All living, breathing, and emotional beings are valuable. It's time we learn how to value ourselves, honor our souls, and take care of our bodies the right way.

Your body is a magnificent creation that houses your eternal soul. Through all of my studies, struggles, heartbreaks, and life experiences, I have learned one critical lesson: My body is the house of God – and so is yours. We were made in God's image, and the kingdom of God lies within us. It's through the mind of the body that we hear the voice of the Holy Spirit. This voice is a tether to God. It is the voice and helper that will fix your life if you let it and when you tap into it. This is not a religious book. This is my philosophy on life and what works for me. I encourage you to come up with an idea that resonates with you and in the meantime read the stories in this book to help you.

You also have an ego. The ego is anything that keeps us judgmental, separated from others, negative, sad, angry, and the list goes on. The ego likes to tell us that we are not good enough, and it makes us question our authority to do and say this or that. The ego likes to play it safe, keep us small, and control everything.

The ego must have a purpose, otherwise, why would we have one? I believe we have an ego so that we can create and make choices. I also believe we have an ego because of duality. We would never know hot if there were no cold. We could never know love if we didn't know hate. It's up to us to choose. We are faced with unlimited options on a daily basis. Are there right and wrong choices, or just choices that do not serve growth?

The Bible, *Conversations with God*, *A Course in Miracles*, and many other spiritual texts say that we are free. We have been given the gift of ultimate freedom to choose what we desire and what we will serve. I believe there is an individualized curriculum for each of our lives. I believe that whatever we are dealing with at any given moment is what we specifically need to learn and grow in order to become a more loving person and help bring us home to who we truly are. I think that we *always* instinctively know what the right choice is. The right choice is the one that is the most loving action for all who are involved – especially you. The right choice will always honor your soul and make you feel good about yourself.

This book is a different kind of self-help, diet, and workout book. It is about the tools (the science of the body) that I have learned, the psychology of the mind, and my philosophy on life. I want to share them with you. You can take what you want and dismiss what does not resonate with you.

I believe that our deepest desire (whether we know it or not) is always to feel the connection with and love of the divine. That is our truest happiness and our very nature. This feeling of peace and love is extremely powerful, and when we are connected to this love, we are completely whole and don't need or want anything outside of ourselves. I believe that many people feel this connection when they fall in love, and that is why we are magnetically drawn to loving relationships. I truly believe that this feeling of love is our natural state. I think it is what heaven is. We can also find this feeling while in meditation or prayer. It completely absorbs us, and we no longer need anything. We experience total bliss. We are in heaven.

Think of the times that you feel completely fulfilled. What are you doing in those moments? If you don't know, start to take notice of the things that fill you up and make you happy and feel fully alive. The process of connecting with the divine is deeply rooted in us. It is like the Earth and Moon's gravity – they go hand in hand. You have a gravitational pull toward feeling this love.

When you are unaware of this pull and not connected to your internal spirit, you will seek fulfillment in relationships (other people), food, a sexy body, a new car, a handbag, fancy shoes, watches, and so on. We are all guilty of seeking fulfillment elsewhere. We often don't even realize we are doing it because it is such a norm in our society. We have been taught to "seek, and ye shall find."

I have looked for fulfillment in relationships, food, and clothing, and it never sustained. On a side note: There is nothing wrong with wanting a nice handbag, a relationship, or beautiful shoes. But if you do not know *who* you are and why you are here, you will suffer, and you will continually look for fulfillment outside yourself.

You will only be fulfilled when you understand that there is a greater meaning to your life and that the most important relationship you have is the one with yourself and the spirit within. When we seek a relationship to give us something that we lack (to complete us), we have chosen wrong. We should come to those things only because they add to whom we are, not because they fill us up or give us something we think we lack.

My definition of our purpose: *To know that we are the holy home of God. God is alive in us (as us) to experience life, receive love, give love, and most of all be love. We are here to remember our purpose through life experiences and grow in love. We can tap into this truth in* *one holy instant. Within a snap of a finger, we can come back home to who we are – God, life, love, and truth. In our pure nature, we are grace. Once we know our purpose, we are to help others obtain this peace as well so that they too can come to understand their purpose and share their light.*

Through the years, I have shifted between things that I thought would make me happy. I have sprinted down paths that I should not have given a second glance, and I have learned a great deal along the way about what I should and should *not* focus on.

The fact is, when we are on our deathbed, the only thing that will matter is how much we loved, who we helped, and what legacy (of love) we left behind.

It took me 36 years to fully embody the message I am about to tell you. Some of those years were filled with excitement and fun, and others were filled with pain, frustration, anger, sleepless nights, and depression. It's funny how life unfolds. It is a great learning lesson, and we must learn the lessons. If we do not learn the lessons, they are bound to show up again.

Why am I telling you all of this? I'm telling you because it all matters. Throughout your entire life, you have been building layers based on the beliefs of your parents, teachers, siblings, co-workers, etc. If those beliefs are out of alignment with your own soul, you will be out of harmony with yourself. You will need to unlearn some things and realign yourself with a life of your own vision and heart beliefs.

I wish that I had this information earlier because I know that it would have saved me much heartache. Many of these lessons, I would not have completely comprehended if they had not fully cracked me open (broken my heart and brought me to my knees) to see a deeper meaning of life and help me see the error of my ways.

What I have come to understand about myself and help others uncover is this message: "I am not a body. I have a body. I am a soul on a mission."

"Am I not a body?" you might wonder. Perhaps you think I am crazy for saying such a thing, but bear with me and let us dive in a little deeper.

We are taught to worship beauty, not the average. We are taught that being different is weird. We are taught that if you don't get married, there is something wrong with you. We are taught that a Barbie (or Superman) body is what we should strive for. We are taught that it is okay to talk negatively about people. We are taught separation, vanity, and fear. We are even taught that we can find the answers through an external God or religion. Then we wonder why we feel lonely and disconnected.

As children, we are not taught healthy self-soothing techniques. The media, religions of the world, and even our parents have taught us that comfort is outside of us because they do not know the truth either. Their elders taught them the same thing. The truth is that you are already perfect just the way you are. You may want things to be different and yes, there is always room for growth, but it is important for you to take your power back and begin to align yourself with your spirit that lives within. You are already whole since the kingdom of God lives within you. Every answer you seek will be revealed to you as you walk your path.

My belief is that all the relationships we seek, we seek because we feel a lack of something, and we wish to fulfill this need. It goes for all relationships: relationships with people, food, sex, love, money, praise, and things – anything that you can attach yourself to. Once it has met our need, we move on unless we are stuck for reasons that we will get into later.

You may love qualities in others that you have not yet cultivated in yourself, and that is something to work towards. But you need nothing outside of you to complete you or to make you better. You have absolute intrinsic value simply because you are *life*.

The second part of the quote I introduced was, "I am free as God created me."

> You cannot walk the world apart from God, because you could not be without Him. He is what your life is. Where you are He is.

There is one life. That life you share with Him. Nothing can be apart from Him and live.[1]

The body is in need of no defense. This cannot be too often emphasized. It will be strong and healthy if the mind does not abuse it by assigning it to roles it cannot fill, to purposes beyond its scope, and to exalted aims, which it cannot accomplish. Such attempts, ridiculous yet deeply cherished, are the sources for the many mad attacks you make upon it. For it seems to fail your hopes, your needs, your values and your dreams.[1]

The body is an amazing home for the Holy Spirit. The body has an incredible ability to heal itself, to feel feelings, to process at speeds faster than any computer, and the list goes on and on. But let us go back for a second and think about the following: If we can't walk the world apart from God, then we can never be apart from God. I love the phrase, "God helps those who help themselves." You cannot sit back and wish and pray for your life to change. You must get up and take action yourself to make things happen.

The following is one of the most empowering and powerful statements you will ever read:

You are responsible for your life. If you're sitting around waiting for someone to save you, to fix you, to even help you, you are wasting your time; because only you have the power to take responsibility to move your life forward. What matters is now, this moment, and your willingness to see this moment for what it is, accept it, forgive the past, take responsibility and move forward. I came to realize, that

---

[1] A Course in Miracles. (2015, June 5). Retrieved July 6, 2015, from http://acim.org/Lessons/lesson.html?daily_lesson=156

all the time I was praying to God asking for God to do something, God was waiting on me.[2]

If we are co-creators with God, we have more power to create (or destroy) our lives than we give ourselves credit for. If the only things that keep us separate from God are our mind, our thoughts, and our ideas of separation, then we have to make sure that we keep our minds holy and on the right path of thought. You do it by putting into action the tools that will keep you aligned with your spirit. Those tools are going to be spelled out here in this book. The Bible also puts a major emphasis on your thoughts:

> Finally, brothers and sisters, whatever is true, whatever is noble, whatever is right, whatever is pure, whatever is lovely, whatever is admirable – if anything is excellent or praiseworthy – think about such things. (Philippians 4:8 New International Version)

Have you ever noticed your energy when you are thinking negative thoughts? It is a dark energy. It drains you and the people around you. Happy thoughts, on the other hand, will always lift you up. "But I can't always be happy," you may be thinking. You are right; things will come up, and they will upset you and make you angry, sad and disappointed. But the good news is you can cultivate a practice that helps you to get out of that dark place *quickly*, and that is of the utmost importance for your happiness on your daily journey. Keep reading because I have outlined tools that will help you.

As an overachiever, I have always set goals and worked very hard at achieving them. Then, once I would succeed, I would wonder, "What's next?"

One day, as I sat and reflected on my life and my achievements, I realized that I barely took time to enjoy life (the journey) because I was

---

[2] Oprah Silenced Her Entire Audience In 44 Seconds with This Life-Changing Statement! I'm Speechless! (n.d.). Retrieved August 13, 2015 from http://www.littlethings.com/oprah-winfrey-44-seconds-video-will-change-your-life/

so focused on the outcomes. That was *not* a healthy way to live, and my life, energy, relationships, and health suffered. I was beginning to realize that the beauty of life happens in the moments and that the most important thing is to enjoy the journey. It's important to love what you do so much that every day, every hour, every minute is honored as the miracle it is. If we are not living a life that glorifies the journey, something needs to change.

So I ask again, are you happy? If not, what would you like to change? Write it down.

I am happy because_____

I am not happy because_____

Instead I would like_____

Know Your Why

Your body is your vessel that must be taken care of. If you do not take care of it, you can rest assured that you will spend countless amounts of hours and money trying to fix it. I have seen it in drones. Many people abuse their bodies with alcohol, food, negative thinking, and neglect. I have done it myself. When I have, I have been prey to sickness, lethargy, and negative self-thinking. I hate being in that place.

I often use the example of a nice car. Who doesn't like or want a shiny, brand new car? We don't want a clunker because that clunker is not going to get us from Point A to Point Z. Your body is the same; if you do not take care of it and feed it the right fuel, it will not get you to your destination in one piece. Just like a vehicle, your body needs to be taken care of.

Having a greater purpose for your life and a huge "why," will make you want to take care of your body. Knowing that you want to leave a massive legacy for your family and the world helps you to stay focused and put the tools into place. Your "why" is more important than you might realize. It's time to write down your mission for this life. Below, write down what you want to do with your life. Make it so big that you have no choice but to take care of your body and mind because your soul longs to do this.

My "why":_____

_____

Client Story: Cindi Fuja

A few months ago, I picked up my daughter from the airport. While we were waiting for her bags, she began to recount a conversation that she and her seatmate had on the flight. The conversation topic was fitness, and my daughter's seatmate was Liz Nierzwicki. Liz had explained the goals and objectives of her new venture and of her dedication to folks who struggle in the areas of health, fitness, and self-awareness. For whatever reason, my daughter's description of Liz's new program (figureFIT!) planted a seed in my brain.

I knew I had to do something to get my health, weight, and stress level under control. I am 55, overweight, and frankly, exhausted most of the time. My dad had a heart attack at age 49 and died. I am sick and tired of being sick and tired. I have more aches and pains than I know what to do with. I. AM. NOT. HEALTHY. And I no longer want to defend that; I want to change it.

I am pretty successful in my professional life. Early on, I realized that I needed to find individuals who I respected or admired and emulate their work ethic and passion for excellence. I would go in early and come home late. I went to professional development workshops and conferences to develop my talents and abilities. Bit by bit, I developed a marketable skill set. I am now the individual that others come to when problems are in need of solutions. I am the one that people come to for advice and questions about best practices.

I am not an unhappy individual, either. I have been married to a wonderful man for 31 years, and I have two compassionate, well-adjusted and professionally successful children. I have a good support network and enjoy getting together with friends. I am fairly certain that when asked, those who know me would describe me as "the fun leader."

The cross I have had to bear most of my life is that I don't have control over my metabolism. Although I was moderately active as a kid (I lived on a farm), I was never comfortable in gym class. I didn't play organized sports, and I always considered myself as "less than" those around me in both coordination and physical ability. That negative self-talk is now a habit. I consistently watch people – not to gain any other information than to determine if I am fatter than the person I am looking at. It is a game I can never win. It does not matter that professionally, personally, and financially, I am at the top of my game. Those things do not matter. What matters is that I hate my physical self. Hate.

Memories are based on what I weighed at the time. I am 5 feet 8 inches tall. At high school graduation, I weighed 135 pounds. My friends weighed between 100 and 110. I only looked at the numbers. I was fat. I weighed 155 when I got married. My bridesmaids had gained weight too, but they were 115 to 125 pounds (and 3 to 4 inches shorter, by the way). It did not matter. I was fat. When I started to think about having kids, I weighed 160 pounds. I went to Weight Watchers and lost 20. Then I gained 40 over the course of the pregnancy. I lost 20 more before baby number two (that is still plus 10 if you are keeping track). I gained 40 more during the pregnancy. I was now close to 200 pounds. I struggled for years going up 10 to 15 then down 15 to 20, and then back up again – always by cutting back on what I ate, or eating the pre-fabricated boxed meals I was getting through NutriSystem or Jenny Craig.

I finally got tired of the roller coaster and just played the part of the jolly fat girl. I did not look in mirrors or get on the scale. I wore knit pants or skirts. I decided to wear black until they developed a darker color. Obviously, I gained weight.

At age 50, I took drastic steps. I got a lap band and lost about 30 pounds overall – mostly because I could not eat that much. I could still eat, however. Crappy food equals crappy results. I plateaued at 200 pounds.

Two years ago, I thought that karma was finally going to help me out. For whatever reason, I started throwing up after every meal. Every meal. While it was disgusting, I started to see results on the scale. Pound after pound. Inch by inch. After six weeks of continued issues, I was down to 165 – my goal weight. I felt like I would finally be happy. But I was not. My hair was stringy and damaged, and I had not had a bowel movement in four weeks. My skin was dull. I felt dizzy more often than not.

Luckily, my husband and kids were noticing. After I had woken up dizzy for the umpteenth time, my husband insisted that I would go to the doctor. He did not give me a chance to say no; he drove me that morning. The doctor took one look at me and told my husband to take me over to St. Joseph Hospital. They admitted me immediately, and after three days, they found out that my lap band had slipped *up* (usually if they slip, it's down), and nothing was getting past the esophagus. My vitamin and mineral levels were so low that the surgeon told me that I was beginning to damage my heart. I had to remove the band rather than fix it.

Fast forward to today. I have gained back all the weight and then some. I am at 235 pounds. Tired. Achy. Fatigued. The words that Liz had told my daughter came to the front of my brain: "I am a fitness and health role model, and I'm helping people learn how to love themselves." Boom. That was it. That was what I needed. If it worked for me in my professional life, why would it not work for me in my fitness life and health? I have never felt that aha moment that everyone who has become fit speaks about, but I think that came pretty darned close. Only three things needed to be done: I had to sign up (easy), tell Liz my story (easier still), and learn what Liz does on a daily basis in terms of fitness, nutrition, and discipline (all hard).

The figureFIT! Program and group community have helped me to see that getting healthy is an everyday activity and a lifelong habit. It is the small choices I make every day that will impact how long and how hard the journey will be.

I am still that person who compares myself to all the fit, thin people walking around – old habits die hard, I guess. What is changing, though, is my outlook. I am beginning to emulate them now rather than compare myself to them. The figureFIT! motto is baby-steps and forgiveness, and I am learning how to do this a little bit at a time. I am cutting my excess carbohydrates. I am stopping the negative self-talk. I am starting (*starting*) to workout.

Join me. It will help both of us. You will not have to worry about being the only heavy person in the program. I will know that I am not the only one who has to gather up the courage to admit that it is okay to have weaknesses. My health and fitness goals can be accomplished by using the same processes I accomplished my professional goals. I have found my fitness role model – my life coach – my guru, in Liz and figureFIT! I am doing this, and I hope you will too.

Cindi Fuja

Age 55

Weight: 233

What to Expect from Reading This Book

Miracles can happen, and it doesn't matter what the struggle looks like – they just happen. It is our mind that thinks our situation is too difficult to change, but there is no order of difficulties in miracles. Think about something that is super easy for you to do. It is easy because you have done it over and over, or maybe it just is easy so there is no question in your mind that you can do it. But when you think of something big like becoming a billionaire or a host of a TV show, be on the cover of Forbes magazine, or own a private jet, you think, "No way. Not me."

Well, I say, "Why not you?" When you prepare yourself for greatness by putting in the daily action steps, things become easier as you walk the path. What is difficult in the beginning becomes easy as you do it over and over again. Something that was once out of the question in your mind becomes like second nature.

"Luck is what happens when preparation meets opportunity." – **Seneca**

I want you to take a moment and open your mind to the possibility that anything can happen in an instant and no matter what your present situation looks like. Happiness lies under all of it, and all you have to do is choose to believe that it is possible.

You may have picked up this book because you were drawn to one or several of the following words: happiness, health, meditation, fitness, or change. We want to get to the root of our psychological issues that are preventing us from moving forward to create real change in our lives. Maybe there is a goal that you want to reach. Maybe there is a habit you are trying to break or even a good habit you are trying to start. Maybe you feel like you are at a turning point in your life, and you are not entirely sure what to do. Maybe you are experiencing depression, anxiety, or some other form of suffering, and you are looking for relief. Maybe you are going through a challenge or recovering from a loss, and you want to find a healthy community to support you in a healthy lifestyle.

Whatever your reason is for wanting change, we all know what it's like to want it. We also all know what it's like to feel stuck when we are trying to change and can't seem to make it happen. We all share the same desire for greater happiness and a greater meaning in our life.

My approach to change is influenced by two traditions: science and spiritual wisdom. Within science is psychology, neuroscience, nutrition science, and exercise science. Within spiritual wisdom is the yoga path, meditation, and the mind-body practices that go along with that tradition.

I studied psychology and nutrition science in college, and I have been training and helping people in this capacity for over 17 years. I have always been particularly interested in understanding how our history makes up our current state of life and how it affects our mindset and health. I am always interested in undoing and taking off the layers that no longer serve us and prevent us from moving forward. Also, knowing this information can help us relieve suffering in our lives. It can help us find a greater sense of happiness and even achieve better health.

Through yoga, I learned that my stress and suffering were part of the influences from my past. The yoga tradition helped me to take off the layers and identify which things were not serving me. As I went through struggles in my life, I began to realize that some of the ideas about life that I was carrying were not mine. They were rather those of my family members or friends I once had close relations to.

In 2014, when I turned away from romantic relationships, I took a deep dive to study myself through a year dedicated to self-love, reading, and meditation. I learned about myself through the practice of meditation, breathing techniques, and through paying attention to and concentrating on certain aspects of my life. As we silence ourselves and turn inwards, much is revealed. All of this helped me to develop personal insight that allowed me to understand myself and what was causing suffering in my life. Slowly I began to change and become much more peaceful and centered.

Between the years of 2011 and 2015, I began to bring together the science and the spiritual path that I had learned to create a program that could support change and healing. Over the years, I have brought this program to my yoga studio, to academic and corporate settings, and to clients all over the world via my online program at figurefitlife.com.

The ideas, insight, science, and wisdom afforded by this program have supported a broad range of changes and transformation in people's lives. Some want to lose weight to improve their physical health. Others wish to overcome anxiety and addictions. Still others long to break free from unhealthy procrastination and perfectionism, or they want to work through negative life scenarios such as abuse or bad relationships.

Whatever your reason is for wanting a change, I hope that my book will offer you a new approach based on self-love and self-compassion, not criticism. It is an approach that uses acceptance and mindfulness as the foundation for changing our inner experiences and our outer actions.

We will walk through three parts that are important to understand in creating the happiest, healthiest, and most fit life. In Part 1, we are going to go over what is our true function on this planet. In my opinion, it is happiness. We were born to be happy. In Part 2, we will talk about our digestive system, health, and nutrition. In Part 3, we will look at how you can exercise for optimum results for your body and mind.

I hope that through both the science and the wisdom, you will learn to trust yourself and your capacity for personal transformation and integrate the tools that are needed to help you live a happy, healthy, and FIT life.

PART 1

HAPPY = Mindset

Happiness Is My Only Job

CHAPTER 1
My Mind is Very Powerful

"Mind is the king of the senses. One who has conquered the mind, senses, passions, thought and reason is a king among men. He is fit for Raja Yoga, the royal union with the Universal Spirit. He has inner light."

– B.K.S. Iyengar

We have all heard that meditation is powerful. Many people say they want to practice meditation but have a difficult time getting started. Others think, "Why should I meditate? I'm just fine the way I am."

I was having a conversation with my client and friend Stacy, and when I started to discuss meditation, it's like her eyes glassed over. I asked her, "why don't you want to meditate?" "I pray. I don't see the point in meditation," was her reply.

Stacy is an amazing, young woman with tons of talent and love for others. She is passionate about fitness and loves working out. There is just one small problem; she struggles with binge eating. I'm very glad she opened up about this negative behavior pattern because it allows me to help her on a deeper level. As we continued our conversation, I asked her, "What if by adding meditation to your life, you never binge ate again? Would you do it?"

"Oh my gosh, yes!" She said.

I explained to Stacy that those bad habits we turn to are simply programmed habits that we have built because, at one point in time, they helped us cope with something. We did it over and over, and it became a habit. However, with concentration, meditation, and knowing what we want for our life, we can break our bad habits and begin to build new ones. Meditation is what helps us to see the whole process unravel and shift our actions so that when we are triggered, we will no longer turn to that same old bad habit.

In this section, I want to talk to you about the science behind meditation and what happens to the brain when we meditate.

The Evaluating Mind and the Experiencing Mind

Each one of us carries the seeds of suffering in our mind. It happens primarily through the human mind's habit of carefully constructing a sense of self that is based on our attitude, our culture, and our personal stories.

Through MRI technology, neuroscientists have discovered that we have two different systems in our brain: the *evaluating* mind and the *experiencing* mind.[3] Depending on which one we are present in, different areas of the brain light up. The evaluation system is our natural state of mind, what we evolved with. It taught us protection, and it taught us how to think critically and make better choices. The experiential system is active when we are concentrating and fully immersed in the present moment.

Take a minute right now to do a mind test. Set a timer for one minute, and during that time sit quietly with your eyes closed, and try not to think about anything. Try to clear your mind.

What happened? Were you able to do it? Did you experience an empty mind? If you are like most people, your mind did not think about

---

[3]   Brain scans show meditation changes minds, increases attention. (2007, June 25). Retrieved August 13, 2015, from http://news. wisc. edu/13890

nothing. In fact, it was probably loaded with thoughts, and you were anything but empty.

The evaluating mind state is always happening unless you are in the present moment (and not off in a story in your thoughts). When you are in the evaluating mind state, you process thoughts in one of four categories.

First, the brain starts to make a *commentary* on what is going on. It tells you things such as "It's cold in here," "I don't like the way that looks," or "that person shouldn't have said that." It is commentating or criticizing something or someone in the present moment. It can also be critical towards itself: "I shouldn't have done this. I'm not doing this right."

Second, in the evaluating state of mind, the brain could be *time traveling*. We go to the past or the future in our thoughts. We relive past experiences and say, "Oh, I should have done this at that moment," or "I should have said this." Or we dream about a future outcome or even fear something happening in our future.

The third thing that happens in the evaluation brain state is what neuroscientists call *self-referential processing*. It interprets what is happening into a sense of who you are. Then it goes to work to build up (or tear down) this sense of self. It labels you and tells you what kind of person you are or are not based on scenarios. For example, if you eat five cookies, it might tell you, "Okay, you ate that fifth cookie. You are not a person who can handle being around cookies." It may also build you up to say things like, "I am the kind of person who does this _____." This process of the brain is talking to you about who you are.

The fourth thing our brain does in the evaluation mode is *social cognition*. When we are in this state, we compare ourselves to others. We say, "This person is more powerful than I am." "This person is not as smart as I am." "This person is ugly, fat (whatever the case may be)." During social cognition, we are building up the self that our brain is creating.

These are the four categories in the evaluation system of the mind. These processes are always happening unless we are concentrating on something in the present moment. Neuroscientists believe this is our natural state of mind and what helped the human race to evolve. It is always active and doing its job even when we are not thinking at all (or trying not to). When you stop concentrating on something or, for example, if you go for a walk, you will find that this is what usually happens with your mind; it becomes very busy.

The yoga tradition says that this state of mind is a large source of our suffering. How can something so natural cause us to suffer? Let's cover each of the four categories of the mind and see how this natural state can cause suffering if we're not careful.

When we are commentating on the environment and constantly thinking that something about the current environment needs to be changed or fixed, it creates dissatisfaction with what is. This constant dissatisfaction deprives the mind of peace in the moment. It prevents us from being present and enjoying the gift of life in the moment. When we are constantly reinforcing this sense of dissatisfaction with what is, we create suffering.

When we time travel, we escape the present moment. Sure, sometimes it's fun to think about the future and dream about things that you wish will happen, and I fully support that when it's done in a very focused way. We will talk about the technique of visualization later in this book. The yoga tradition teaches us that no experience is fully improved by escaping it.

When the mind builds up this sense of self, it is constantly telling us who we are, what makes us feel comfortable, what makes us uncomfortable, etc. When we do this, it distances us from others and creates a rigid sense of rules as to how things should be. The fact is that change is always happening. When we fight change, and the self that we have built can't adapt, we suffer. For example, say someone challenges you or criticizes you, or you experience rejection or fail at something. Then you may feel like something is wrong with you, or you will defend this sense of self that you have created. If you embody the fact that something is wrong with "you," you may think that you are incapable of change.

The evaluating mind is a productive state of mind. It has helped us to be creative, protect ourselves from harm, and plan for what to do if and when something happens. But when there is nothing to protect against and no reason to be solving an imagined problem, it can be a big source of suffering.

Neuroscientists have found that meditation is a powerful practice that helps us strengthen the alternative mind called the "experiencing mind." However, the active evaluating mind makes people believe that they will never be able to meditate because they can't slow down the mind. This lack of knowledge about the brain keeps them from experiencing one of the greatest benefits known to mankind. The truth is everybody's mind is active like this unless trained or engrossed in a task. With knowledge comes power. Now that you know what the brain is doing and *how* to help it, you will be able to learn how meditate and experience the great peace that can only come from this powerful practice.

Neuroscientists were only able to discover this alternate (experiencing) state of mind by studying the brains of meditators. They found that the parts of the brain that process present moment awareness, such as sight, sound, smell, touch, taste, and feelings, were larger (thicker gray matter) and had more connections between the neurons than in the brains of non-meditators. They also found that the meditators were able to stay in the experiencing mind longer than non-meditators, essentially creating a new normal state of mind.

Results of Meditation

*"Gratitude connects me to spirit." – **Liz Nierzwicki***

How amazing that the ancient yoga tradition knew all along that we could change this natural state of mind through the practice of concentrating. With concentration comes meditation. And via meditation, we slow down the mind and gain peace, clarity, and wisdom. The yogis discovered the peace of a quiet mind and realized that an active mind could be a big source of suffering. They realized that when we are in a state of mind that is always trying to change reality, constantly unsatisfied, and looking for something wrong, it's no wonder why there is no peace.

One day, a client, Amanda, told me about a guy she had met the day before. She was excited about meeting him and had an instant crush about the possibilities of a relationship with him. She was going on and on about how they were so compatible. In her mind, she was already walking down the isle with this man.

I told her, "You know, Amanda, I understand your excitement for this guy, but you are delusional about him."

She looked at me with huge eyes. "I am?" She came closer and plopped her head on her chin.

"Think about it... what is reality offering you? Is he calling you? Is he asking you out?" I asked.

"No, he's not," she answered.

I was not trying to discourage her. I was just trying to get her to see how the mind works when it wants something. The mind is strong; it creates stories and situations. If we are not careful, we jump on the crazy train and ride the train all the way to crazy town getting caught up in the stories.

We continued our conversation, and I said, "It's okay to dream and envision your future. In fact, I encourage it through visualization. Just make sure that you're not making yourself miserable by building up this person in your head, imagining walking down the aisle, and creating an imaginary life that reality is not backing up. That only leads to disappointment, and then you wonder why things are not happening. When you find yourself doing this, Amanda, just do anything to get yourself back to the present moment and what is really happening. Find something to be grateful for, and do something that *you* enjoy to help you lift your energy. You may or may not end up going out with this man, but don't let yourself get so wrapped up in this story that if it does not happen, you will be sad. Do not give anyone that much power over you. Be your own booster, and go do something that you enjoy. Life will open up to you as it is supposed to. I know it's easier said than done when emotions are involved, but it is so important to have this awareness."

The next day, she told me that our conversation had helped her tremendously. She had realized that many of her disappointments in life were due to imagined scenarios, good and bad, which were only stories in her head.

Once I started to practice present moment awareness via meditations, I started to realized the many different lives and stories going on in my head. The things our mind will tell us and the stories it will create are quite amazing.

The practice of meditation does two things. First, it helps you to see where your mind is going when it is in the evaluating mode of thinking. You become aware of how often you travel to stories of the past or visions of grandeur (or fears) in the future. You're able to see when you become a critic. You see when you are creating a self and building that self up with, "I am the type of person who does this or doesn't do that." And you see when you are comparing yourself to others.

Second, meditation strengthens this part of your brain. As a muscle is strengthened when you lift weights, this area of the brain can get stronger and grow bigger as well. So when you notice yourself in the evaluating state of mind, you can, in an instant, switch to something in the present moment and hold your concentration here to keep you in the present. Keep your focus on things that you see, smell, hear, and feel. Move into the sensations of the present moment, give gratitude for life, and tune into your breath.

I find that the practice of meditation and remaining in the present moment (rather than in your head) is becoming more critical to our health and happiness than ever before. We simply have too many distractions in modern society – too many things wanting our attention. If we do not know how to turn off and tune in, then happiness, peace of mind, and clarity of our purpose will elude us.

The practice of being mindful of the present moment helps you to notice your breath, energy, and feelings. It also helps you move into the sensations going on within you. You become much more aware of everything going on around you *and* within you. This cannot be underestimated. We often hear the phrase, "trust your gut instincts," but if you are so out of tune with yourself, you will not hear your spirit's urgings until it's too late, and you find yourself on your knees praying for something to change.

The wonderful news is that neuroscientists have discovered that meditation is like a workout for your brain. It can help you to create and grow this "new" default experiencing or mindful state of mind. With as little as eight weeks of mindfulness and concentration meditation training, you can begin to strengthen this part of your brain.[4] With practice, you will become better and better at noticing when you slip off into doing one of the four evaluating behaviors and bring yourself back. And with practice, the experiential system, rather than the evaluation system, slowly begins to become your default state of mind.

Experienced meditators are aware of what the mind is doing. During my one-year deep dive into learning about myself, I found that the more I practiced meditation, the better I could see where my mind was going when drifting out of the present moment. "Oh, there it goes to that old story again," or, "Why am I thinking of that now?" It's interesting what an uncontrolled mind does and the stories it tells us.

When I first started meditating, one of my first experiences realizing my mind's wanderings was when I was going through a breakup. As I was getting ready one day in the bathroom, putting on my eye makeup, it hit me like a ton of bricks; my mind was riding the crazy

---

[4] Brain scans show meditation changes minds, increases attention. (2007, June 25). Retrieved August 13, 2015, from http://news. wisc. edu/13890

train of thoughts. I was telling myself stories about my ex. I was in the evaluating mind and I was time traveling. I was imagining completely made up scenarios, and I had no idea whether they were true or not. I was riding the crazy train to my imagined truth of these stories, and my energy was reflective of this negative story I was telling myself. I felt it.

Then I stopped dead in my tracks, looked myself square in the eye, and said, "You're delusional right now." It was like I stepped out of myself and saw myself. I laughed at the realization of what I was doing. I saw what I was doing and was thrilled to be able to bring myself back to the present. I said, "I see you, but I choose to think positive thoughts instead." Then I completely stopped the thoughts dead in their tracks.

My one-year deep dive into meditation and concentrating on me, my life, and my habits was the best year of my life in terms of understanding the peace of God living within me. I began to realize more and more that I am not my mind. I am the conscious chooser, and only what I choose to focus on is what I will create for myself.

Now that you know the neuroscience behind the mind, you can find rest knowing that you are normal. Whew! And your kids are normal. The mind is meant to be active. It is going to do what it does, and that is think, think, think. It is our job to tame it with activities that will help us do so.

The Course in Miracles states: "Your mind is dividing its allegiance between two kingdoms." It's beautiful that meditation allows you to train your mind to become the master of it. With continued practice of meditation, you can recover more quickly from the distractions of your default mind and consciously return to your current experience. As you spend less time in the default state, you will strengthen the regions of the brain that process the current moment. That allows you to grow this region and system of the brain and, therefore, get better at staying in the present moment.

Meditation helps you become an observer of your mind and see what the mind does. You are not your mind or your thoughts. You are the spirit that lives within. The great news is that you get to choose what you think about. This awareness gives you space to move away from the evaluation system and bring your mind back into the experiencing system in the moment. As you direct the brain to come back to the present moment, you will strengthen this system and become more self-aware.

It's my belief that when we are in the present moment, we are literally in God. When we drift off into the webs of the mind, we begin to create or construct things that may or may not be beneficial based on our guiding system. When we give ourselves over to the spirit to lead, we are open to the beauty, love, and life that is always present to us in the moment. When we let the ego lead, we are left with confusion, anger, distrust, etc.

I find that when I start to worry about my business or whether something is going to turn out a certain way, I get stressed. I remind myself of this passage in the Bible:

> Therefore, I tell you, do not worry about your life, what you will eat or drink; or about your body, what you will wear. Is not life more than food, and the body more than clothes? Look at the birds of the air; they do not sow or reap or store away in barns, and yet your heavenly Father feeds them. Are you not much more valuable than they? Can anyone of you by worrying add a single hour to your life? And why do you worry about clothes. So do not worry, saying, 'What shall we eat?' or 'What shall we drink?' or 'What shall we wear?' [Y]our heavenly Father knows that you need them. But seek first his kingdom and his righteousness, and all these things will be given to you as well. Therefore, do not worry about tomorrow, for tomorrow will worry about itself. Each day has enough trouble of its own. (Matthew 6:25-34 New International Version)

It's easy to get caught up in the stories we tell ourselves and create stress and suffering. Think about a thought that has triggered you to act or react a certain way. What was the thought? What happened in your body? When we accept a thought and latch on to it, we embrace the hormones and chemical response in the body that the thought will bring. Thoughts are powerful, and they create in some way shape or form always, even if that is only via your feelings.

Beliefs come from past experiences.

Emotions are anchors to the past.

When we have thought the same thoughts over and over, we create beliefs. A belief is created by nothing more than replaying of an old thought or emotion about something from the past. When you think the same thoughts over and over again, the body becomes subconsciously programmed to replay the same neurological response pattern over and over again. As a result, it keeps you doing exactly the same things and feeling the exact same way. If we want to change a belief, we have to make a firm decision to create a new thought that will bring a new energetic pattern. Then when we have a different behavior. We will move our brain and body out of the past and into the present moment, allowing us to create a different experience.

*"If you do not go within, you go without." – **Neale D. Walsch***

Meditation allows us to look at the habits of the mind. When we can see what the mind is doing, we can free ourselves from the emotions and attachments that get brought up. We free ourselves from the thoughts and emotions by looking directly at the thoughts and seeing them as what they are – a thought that has no power over us. We can, therefore, use meditation to help us transform our experiences.

Life is happening in the moment. When we learn to rest our body and mind in the present moment, not judging or grasping thoughts, we are supported by the newness the present experience provides. When we rest in our organic human nature of peace, joy, love, and wisdom, we can be healed. All we have to do is choose to be in the present in the experience of the moment rather than in the mind of the evaluating system.

Some of my clients tell me that they can't meditate because they can't slow down their mind. Once I teach them about the two systems of the brain, and they experience witnessing it for the first time, they become surprisingly excited. They begin to see the light at the end of the tunnel. I let them know that it is not a problem that the mind wanders because it's the mind's job to think. I help them to see that it is not a failure when the mind wanders in meditation because this is the learning process. It helps us to see what the mind is doing so that we can control it instead of being controlled by it. The important thing to do when it happens is to refocus the mind on something in your present environment.

I have a simple process that I follow when I notice my mind wandering. I call it my "Holy Instant Meditation." In a holy instant, I am home to my spirit with a simple refocusing of the mind.

Holy Instant Meditation:

1. Become *aware* of what the mind is doing.

2. *Forgive* the thought. The worst thing we can do is being hard on our self for something that is natural – thinking. Just because we are thinking a thought doesn't mean we need to keep our focus on that thought.

3. *Refocus* on something in the present moment, particularly something positive that you can offer gratitude for.

4. Offer *gratitude* for your new self-awareness and know that you are getting better at living in the present moment.

With the information from neuroscientists and the yoga tradition, I have come up with a chart to help identify the nature of the mind. Due to the nature of the mind, we are either asleep or awake, and when we are operating under a specific guiding system, we are doing the following:

Awake Mind	Asleep Mind
Spirit	Ego
Love	Hate
Experiencing Mind	Evaluating Mind
Truth/Reality	Illusions/Perceptions
Heaven	Hell

Empowering Thought	Fearful Thought
Resurrection	Crucifixion
Union/Connectedness	Separation
Joy, Happiness, etc.	Judgment, Hate, etc.
Sanity	Insanity
Abundance	Scarcity/Loss

I use this visualization in my workshops as a teaching tool to help people understand their mind better. When we begin to understand how our mind works, we can understand that we are not our mind. We are the observer of our mind, and in a holy instant, we have the choice to bring our thoughts back to an awake mind.

Understand Your Mind, Understand Your Life?

"We will not recognize what we receive until we give it. Whatever is lacking is because you are not giving it" – *A Course in Miracles.*

Each thought you have creates the experience of your life. If you do not like the situations in your life, it is time to take a look back at your thoughts and subsequent actions that have created your life.

Do you believe that people are helpful or that they can't be trusted? Whichever one you believe is what the Universe will give you because the Universe always wants to support your true belief.

I believe we are *all* doing the best we can with what we know in each moment. If we knew more, we would make better choices. Every experience in your life is a lesson to help you be the best you that you can be. As children, we learn about life from those around us and our inner feelings. We have layers added to our beliefs by those we lived with or spent time with as we grew up. This is what we know until we decide to lose those layers. We will recreate how we know to react. We treat ourselves the way our parents treated us. We love ourselves the same way our parents loved us.

It is easy to blame our parents for where we are in life. But remember that your parents were doing the best they could with the intellect and knowledge they had. Instead of blaming them, try to understand them. Figure out what their childhood looked like. How did their parents treat them? If they were not shown love as children, they wouldn't know how to show love to you. Take yourself out of the mode of victim and dive into an empathetic mindset that will help you to see where they may have been broken and never received healing.

The cycle must be broken somewhere if anything is going to change. The Universe has delivered this book to you for a reason. You are on a mission of learning to love yourself, and this will change the trajectory of your life as well as the lives of your children and grandchildren. The change will come all because you took the time to learn how to love yourself. When you know how to love yourself, then you will know what you deserve, and you will know how to treat people.

Life is about thoughts. Each moment, the only thing you deal with is a thought and the feeling associated with that thought. We think thoughts about ourselves, our job, our finances, other people, etc. When you become aware of your thoughts, you will begin to have more power and control over your life.

If you allow yourself to be a victim of your mind's wanderings, you will be a victim of those thoughts. Your power is in the present moment and in knowing what you are thinking.

When you are unhappy with your body or your life, it is likely that you are dealing with a bit (or a lot) of self-hatred. If you have negative feelings about yourself, change the thought, and the feelings will go away as well. I like to tell my clients that thoughts such as, "I am not good enough," "They are better than me," and "I'm not ready" are from the ego. The ego mind will tell you that you're not good enough, not ready, and nobody will care about what you have to say. Don't believe the ego. We may have the same thoughts over and over. It is important to recognize them as habits of the mind that can be changed by thinking new thoughts that empower you.

Consistency is the biggest determinant of the success of any goal you want to achieve: weight loss, positive self-talk, money making, etc. If you have found that you tend to speak negatively about yourself or your life, then you will have to put into practice forgiveness. Start forgiving yourself every time a negative thought comes up. Switch it over to one you want to think, and then keep up this practice until it becomes a new habit.

Whatever is happening "out there" is only a mirror of what is going on inside of you. We attract what we think about ourselves. When we believe that we are not good enough, we will attract people into our lives that reinforce that thought. The good news is that when you no longer think this way, those people go away. We rise above anyone or anything that will treat us like less than we know we deserve. Instead, we start to attract those of a different energetic level. Energy always finds like energy.

All resentment, blame, and guilt are like cancer in your body and are sources of disease. When we are ill, we need to search our heart for any resentment towards anybody. We must forgive them so that any resentment can be dissolved.

When clients come to me, the first thing I work on with them is their mind and helping them understand what it is doing. I focus here because if there is no self-awareness of the operating system of the mind, nothing else will fall into place. I want my clients to understand the power of the mind and use it effectively to find peace and understanding in their life. The second thing I work on with clients is teaching them that they are worthy of their own attention. If they are not happy with themselves, they will not be happy with anyone else.

The power of meditation in your life is beyond measure; this is why I have included meditation in my program. Meditation is the most powerful transformation tool that we have available to us, and it's free! When we understand our mind, what it is doing, and the stories it is telling us, we can start to reel it in. Then we become the controller of our thoughts and, therefore, our life.

Starting on Your Meditation Journey

Meditation is fairly easy now that you know how the brain works. You now know that when your mind wanders, it is only doing its job. Your job as the observer is to bring it back to the present moment. It becomes easy with practice. I recommend that you dedicate some time to meditation every morning, whether it be 5 minutes or 20 minutes, just make it happen.

Begin by sitting down in an area where you are free from distractions. Do not lie down because if you lie down, you might fall asleep. Find a comfortable position and just sit with yourself, the moment, your breath. You don't need music. Start following your breath. Inhale through the nose and exhale through the mouth.

When the mind starts to wander off, bring it back to your breath. You might have to do that 30 times, and that is okay. I sometimes give people something to focus on in the beginning. It could be a mantra (a repeated phrase), such as "I" (on the inhale) and "am" (on the exhale). Or it could be an image of something like a beach or their favorite place. When you sit down to meditate, you can simply focus on your breath and then align your mind with the image of a beach or somewhere that gives you happiness. When your thoughts go off track, which they inevitably will do, then bring it back with compassion. Bring your mind back to the thought, the mantra, or the image in your mind. You could set a timer. As soon as the timer goes off, you can stop meditating.

You might want to have a journal handy when your meditation is over. There might be insights, something that you learned, something that you felt, or something that came up during your meditation that you want to write down. I have post-it notes and reminders all over the place to remind me of the powerful insights that have come through for me during meditation. Trust what comes up for you and know that you are experiencing exactly what you need to be experiencing in the moment. With daily practice, meditation gets easier. The times when your mind pulls you off into the evaluation state become fewer and farther between.

The mind begins to process much more slowly, and you begin to have space between your thoughts. This space is sometimes called pure consciousness or our alignment with the divine. This is the place where we have the potential to hear our internal divine spirit talk to us, guide us, and help explain life to us.

"There is a voice that doesn't use words. Listen." – **Rumi**

This voice is the seat of our soul, our intuition, or spirit. The voice of our soul becomes increasingly louder with continued practice of listening to it.

Meditation affects many different aspects of our life. It affects our mental state, our physical state, our relational state, and our environmental state. Meditation answers the main question in life: Who am I? When you begin to meditate, when you begin to slow down, you begin to realize the answers to that question.

CHAPTER 2
Self-Love

The secret to happiness is always loving yourself and knowing that you are completely whole on your own without external approval or attachments.

– Liz Nierzwicki

What is self-love? Have you ever taken the time to cultivate a deep love for yourself, your unique feelings, and all of your life experiences that made you who you are? To fully understand yourself and why you do what you do, I believe it's important to take the time to honor your heart and what it has been through. Honor your experiences. Honor why you felt the way you did in certain situations and why you made a specific decision (perhaps because your intuition knew). Honor your relationships, heartaches, and choices, and look back to see what served you and what did not. From this place of understanding, you can reach out to yourself with love and support.

It is easy to value the wrong things when we are taught to think that happiness is "out there." We put Band-Aids on our brokenness with shiny new things. However, that does not serve us and it never will. The only thing that will help you is to stop and take a deep look at yourself. Consider how you treat yourself, how you love yourself, and the choices you have made and continue to make. From that place of awareness, you learn about yourself. Then you begin to make choices about how to move forward honoring yourself and creating the best life that you can create.

Loving yourself means to be your own best friend. Loving yourself means that you do not betray yourself. Loving yourself means only choosing situations and relationships that honor your divinity and respect your body. Loving yourself means eating foods that are healthy because you want to treat your body well. Loving yourself mean you talk kindly to yourself after you have made a mistake because you realize that you are human and that we all make mistakes. Loving yourself means exercising because you want to protect your body and keep it as a well-tuned optimally working machine. People who love themselves do not abuse themselves because they want to treat their holy home with love and respect.

How do you know when you love yourself? You love yourself when you can truly be yourself and are not worried about being judged by others. Only you know who you are and what you have been through to make you that person, so other people's judgment doesn't matter. You will know that you love yourself when you do not lose yourself in love, work, or other things. You love yourself when your honor your spirit and what it is telling you and you make choices that serve you rather than harm you.

Your life is on a highly individualized path towards enlightenment about who you are and help you understand your incredible capabilities to create a magnificent life for yourself. All of what you have gone through in your life has had a purpose of teaching you something and help you grow into the unique person you are meant to be. When you realize the power of letting go of the past and embrace your power in the present moment, you become unstoppable.

When someone knows what self-love is, they acknowledge their intuition, energy, and feelings. Loving yourself means to honor your sensitivity and understanding that it is there to tell you something.

Take a moment to answer these questions:

- What is going on in your life?

- How is your health?

- Do you like your work?

- How are your finances?

- How did your last relationship end?

After you answer the questions, ask yourself about your beliefs behind each of those questions. What do you believe to be true for you? Once you answer that, sit in meditation asking yourself if you are limiting yourself by your beliefs.

Now take a moment to talk about your parents. My parents:

_____

_____

_____

Now fill out this section:

I should:

_____

_____

Why?

_____

_____

I should:

_____

_____

Why?

_____

_____

I should:

_____

_____

Why?

_____

_____

Take a look at all the "shoulds" and "whys" you just mentioned, and ask yourself if that is something that *you* want to do. Is it truly a deep calling in your heart, or is it something that someone else wants you to do or thinks you should do?

It's important that you learn how to separate yourself from the things you want in your life versus what others want from your life. Many parents, sisters, brothers, friends, spouses, etc., project onto you what they think you should do based on their perception of your life. But their perception of your life is skewed because they do not know your full truth or your heart's desires. Even as well as someone may know you, they are still not you, and they do not know what is best for you; only you do.

Your power comes from taking back your life and setting a path for yourself based on what *you* want to do. Remember that it's not out there. No one has the answers for you. Only you can search your heart and make the appropriate choices. I believe we all have an image in our mind of who we want to be. By taking consistent action toward your dreams and goals, you create a wonderful life that honors you and everyone you come in contact with. So what do *you* want?

Let's replace the "shoulds" with this phrase: "If I desire to, I will":

_____

_____

If I desire to, I will

_____

_____

If I desire to, I will

_____

_____

If I desire to, I will

_____

_____

If I desire to, I will

_____

_____

If I desire to, I will

_____

_____

Know that just because life is saying no to you right now, it doesn't mean that it is saying no to you forever. The Universe has a miraculous way of working all things in your favor when you continuously strive towards the things you desire. When there is a no in your life, say thank you because that only means there is something better lined up than what you envisioned. I know that's a tough one to embody, especially when you have set your heart and soul on something. I promise that as you get closer to your soul or spirit during meditation, you will begin to see life much more clearly, and you will begin to be grateful for everything life has delivered to you. It's only through the process of forgiveness that our load is lightened, and we move into a state of gratitude.

Take back your power and do things that make you happy. When you are happy doing the things that *you* want to do, you will have the ultimate power over your life. You will no longer be able to blame or resent others because you are the one making the choices in your life.

I see it in my own family, in my clients, and at work with my employees, people blaming others for why things are or are not happening in their own lives. Yes, there are certain times you may be waiting for something from someone else, but you always have a choice in every situation, even if that choice means you will no longer wait for someone else to get something done in order for you to move forward.

Watch where and when you play the victim. Hint: Anytime you play the victim card, you blame someone else for something they did to you. When you notice that you blame others, take a moment to *stop* and think about where you added to the situation or problem. Then take responsibility for your side of the street. It can be easy to blame others and say, "You did this to me."

Instead take a look at your behavior – everything you co-created with the other person. Then take responsibility for your side. If you look honestly, you will find that nothing was done to you that you did not ask for in some way, shape, or form. (Obviously, this excludes things that happened to you as a child.) How can you *stop* blaming others and take your power back right here, right now?

Judgment or criticism is another form of victim mentality. When we judge others, we think we know how things should be. But the truth is we don't know the other person's life, what makes that person who they are, or what they have been through. Judging is a bad habit that will keep you in a small-minded box.

The Course in Miracles says the following about judgment:

> Remember how many times you thought you knew all the "facts" you needed for judgment, and how wrong you were! Is there anyone who has not had this experience? Would you know how many times you merely thought you were right, without ever realizing you were wrong? Why would you choose such an arbitrary basis for decision-making? Wisdom is not judgment; it is the relinquishment of judgment.[5]

Let go of your judgment of others and theirs of you. Forgiveness is key if you feel like you have been wrongly judged by others. The key is letting go and letting the moment heal you. Remember your power is always in the present moment.

What Do You Love?

Here is a list of some of the things I am grateful for:

- Life and being alive

- My family

- Freedom

- My home

- The Internet to learn and work from

- Peacefulness

- Healthy foods

- Mobility – the freedom to move my body, drive, and fly places

- The Universe

---

[5] 10. How Is Judgment Relinquished? (n.d.). Retrieved August 13, 2015, from http://www.jcim.net/acim_us/MNL-10.php

Name some things you love:

_____

_____

_____

_____

_____

_____

What are some ways that you do not love yourself?

_____

_____

_____

_____

_____

_____

Here are some ways that I have been unloving towards myself:

- I have not been careful with my heart.

- I have mistreated my body with food.

- I have procrastinated doing things that were not important.

- I have let people stay in my life too long when I knew I needed to say goodbye to them.

- I have spoken negatively to myself.

- I have not honored my intuition.

- I have not honored the energy my body was giving me around certain people.

When we focus on the things we love about life, we will get more to be grateful for. Know that you have the option of observing things as they are or imagining them the way you would like them to be. Know that whichever option you choose, your thoughts will produce an energetic vibration within you that will draw events and circumstances to you that match this vibration. If you do not like where you are, go out and put yourself into an action that will bring the feeling you want to manifest.

Think – Do – Be

Think about what you want.

Go **do** things that will bring you what you want.

Be in the experience of what you want.

When we do this over and over, we will create the life that we want. This is our true power.

CHAPTER 3
I'm Taking My Power Back

To become happy, it's important to practice and cultivate happiness in your daily life. For a quantum shift to happen, you need to change the way you think about reaching your goals. You can make all the goals you want, but if you don't understand where you sabotage yourself, you will not move forward.

We do not guard our thoughts enough. Our thoughts are incredibly powerful, so we need to be careful with what we are thinking. Thoughts become things, so we must focus the mind on the positive. It's important to become aware of the stories we tell ourselves. We often hold on to something someone said about us, and we make it true for ourselves. We must let go of those stories and embrace our truth.

What have you held on to because of someone else's idea of who you are? Take a minute to think about all the things you tell yourself about why you can't have the body, job, or the life you want. Take a moment to write down your limiting beliefs about yourself.

I believe I can't have _____

because of _____.

I believe I can't have _____

because of _____.

I believe I can't have_____

because of _____.

People often come to me with excuses. Although they do not see the stories they tell as excuses, they are. They become to wrapped up in the stories they tell themselves that they feel as if they are facts. I often hear people say that they could never eat a certain way or take the time to do workouts or food preparation. When I hear such excuses, I want to grab the ones who said them and shake those thoughts right out of their head because these thoughts and words shape their life and keep them stuck. They want change. However, they are so comfortable where they are that they are not willing to take the steps to change their life and patterns to suit a new goal.

If somebody says, "I don't have time," they will never have time because they are not willing to make the time. The fact is that we make time for what we want. If someone really wants change, they will begin to get uncomfortable because a short time of discomfort can change their life forever.

We do not grow when we stay inside our comfort zone. I set a reminder on my phone to remind me to "Get uncomfortable." When it goes off, I do something that is out of my comfort zone, like email the *Oprah Winfrey Show* a video of my keynote presentation. Why? Because the only way we get what we want is by going after it.

Limiting Beliefs

We will always get what we seek, think, and talk about. Thinking "I could never do that" or "I do not have the time for that" are examples of what I call limiting beliefs. People need to recognize these stories that they tell themselves and begin to tell themselves new stories.

I was talking to a friend at dinner, and we were discussing how you get what you think. He said, "It's like driving a motorcycle. You are taught to look exactly where you want your bike to turn because you will drive wherever you look. If you see a car on the side of the road and you're looking at the car while you're turning the motorcycle, you will drive right into the car. You must look where you want to go."

We need to cultivate our awareness of our thoughts and especially our limiting beliefs. The figureFIT! Worksheet I: "Acknowledge Your Limiting Beliefs" in the Appendix will help you identify which limiting beliefs you have.

What I usually see behind a limiting belief is a negative thought about oneself, rooted in fear. It can be thoughts such as "I'm not good enough," "People don't like me," or "I'm afraid of rejection." Or it could be "I will never be that pretty," "I could never be that fit because my body is not made to be that thin or fit," or "How come everybody else has such a great body and I don't?" These are all limiting beliefs. Unless we start telling ourselves a new story *and* start to change our actions, these beliefs will keep us stuck. Nothing changes until we start to do something differently. We *must* change the way we think, talk, act, and react.

Have you ever sat down and looked at all the stories you tell yourself? Take a moment to sit and write a stream of consciousness regarding your fears and all the reason you think you can't have what you want. Then write another stream of consciousness to uncover why you think you have those fears. In the end, you might say that you do not feel loved. That is the place where you shatter your limiting beliefs and tell yourself a new story. If your limiting belief is "I don't think people like me," then write a new affirmation such as "I have many friends who love me," and "I am lovable."

The key to moving past limiting beliefs is to begin to do things that you love and make you feel alive. Affirm yourself by saying your new thoughts out loud multiple times a day when the old stories come up.

I like to say the opposite of whatever thought pops into my head. For example, I'll say, "I don't believe this. I believe _____." (Fill in the blank with a new affirmation).

We can't change our beliefs until we realize and recognize that they are not helping us but only holding us back. You can say, "I see this old belief as something I no longer choose to think about, and I choose to see my life differently."

For every limiting belief, think of a new story that you will tell yourself when it comes up. You need to bridge the gap between where you are and where you want to go with your thoughts. You can't go from saying, "I'm fat" to saying "I'm a supermodel." You won't believe it, so you have to bridge the gap. You could say, "I am making the best choices to give me the best and healthiest body." And as you do the workouts, that is the truth, and you can support the thought with the feelings. Always make the new affirmation in the present tense and take a walk with your actions and thoughts to get you to where you want to be.

Thoughts are powerful – yes! But you can't just sit around and think; you must also act. So act like an athlete. Be a fit person *now*. When you are at a restaurant, order the food that a fit person would eat. Exercise like a fit person. Say "No, thank you" to desserts like a fit person would, and soon you will be the fit person.

The Downward Spiral of Negative Thoughts

One morning in 2009, I was trying on some clothes before work, and they were too tight for me. At the time, I was not prioritizing fitness; I let everything else get in front of my workout time. Since the clothes I had put on were tight, I had to find something bigger to wear, but I had nothing. My entire wardrobe was too small for me, and I did not want to go spend money to buy larger clothes. I was mad.

It was a moment of anger and self-criticism. I was telling myself "Liz, you're so fing fat that it is ridiculous." I spoke to myself in a way that nobody would want to be spoken to. A wave of negative feelings swept over me. My thoughts, words, and energy were all destructive. In my mind flashed a downward spiral, and I knew my spirit was telling me, "*Stop!* This is where you're going with this belief." Then I suddenly realized that my way of talking to myself was taking me down that spiral. I stopped my words and sat in the feeling for a second.

At that moment, I decided that I had to change my thoughts and the way that I talked to myself. I needed to find a better way to motivate myself. Rather than beating up myself with my thoughts and word, I had to find a way to uplift myself.

The following weeks, I continued thinking about how to uplift myself. I started looking for quotes that made me happy, and I wrote them down. I pulled out some fitness magazine covers that illustrated what I aspired to do and be, and I hung these up so that I had something in front of me to motivate me and keep me on track.

I began to realize that I had to tell myself a new story and couldn't talk to myself like I had been. I realized that the feelings I was having were not serving me, and I was the only one who could change the way I felt. I was the only one who could put in the work in the gym and eat the right foods so that I would never feel like that again.

Over the next weeks and months, I began establishing a new habit. When words such as "I'm not good enough," "I'm fat," or "I'm never going to have this" came up in my head, I would immediately switch over my thoughts to something positive. I would start thinking about something that I had power over. If I said, "I'm sick and tired of being fat," I would immediately stop myself and say "I am doing everything in my power to be the best and healthiest version of me." I switched it over into a more affirmative and empowering thought. That simple step changed my energy along with my actions. It led me down a path that helped me start living the way that I wanted to live and do what I needed to do to get where I wanted to be.

I started cultivating new ways of dealing with my negative stories and feelings. Then I started to teach these new ways to my clients, and they began benefiting from them. These new ways were as follows:

1. I became *aware* of the negative things that I was saying to myself.

2. I *forgave* myself for the thoughts or stories. Then I wrote them down and realized that it was not me; it was just thoughts.

3. I *switched* the dialog to something that I had power over and something that made me feel better.

4. I *affirmed* this new story with notes, reminders on my phone, gratitude, and journaling.

What I came to learn was that when we have limiting beliefs, or when we tell ourselves something negative, we call that into our lives. The perfect example is the person who is always thinking that their spouse (or significant other) will cheat on them. It happens because their gut already told them that it was going to happen. It is called the Law of Attraction.

The Law of Attraction says that what you say, what you think, and what you feel, you manifest in your life. I believe that this is precisely how we create our lives.

After my closet experience in 2009, I did a lot of work on my thoughts through meditation. I reflected on my past to see what thoughts I had about life, what choices I made based on these thoughts, and where those choices led me. I realized that my entire life was my creation. People came and went along my path, and they helped or hindered me, but the Universe gave me exactly what I called upon.

I encourage you to reflect on your beliefs about yourself, the people around you, and life itself. Then begin to notice the thoughts you have regarding those things. Your thoughts lead to actions, and those actions lead to the life you create. If you do not like where you are, it's time to think new thoughts that will result in new actions. Follow the four-step process above to help change any area of your life. It is an extremely powerful process, and if you are ready to change your life, do not delay another day. To make this process even more powerful, write down your limiting beliefs above and then the new stories (and subsequent actions) you will tell yourself.

In the figureFIT! community, I encourage the members and private coaching clients to share their stories and limiting beliefs with each other in order to get them out of their mind, take the power away from them, and overcome them. Limiting beliefs only keep us stuck. As they identify the stories and begin to do the work that is needed, they begin to transform into the person they always knew they could be. It is wonderful to see people learn how to love themselves and bloom into beautiful, fully alive human beings who love life.

When we tell ourselves a negative story, such as "I'm stupid," "I'm fat," or "I will never have this," we will manifest exactly those things. It is imperative that we stop the thought immediately and say out loud the exact opposite thing.

Saying something out loud gives power and energy to the words. Don't just say something out loud once; repeat it for about 90 seconds. In the book *Hardwired Happiness*, the author Rick Hanson states that if we want to keep something in our experience and let it dig roots, we must think about that thing for a minimum of 60 seconds. By doing so, you will begin to hardwire this new thought into your idea and belief about yourself. This is the first step of calling in the life you wish for.

Limiting beliefs will never fully go away, but you will get better and better at noticing them, and you learn that they have power *if and only if* you believe them. Our job is to become aware of what we are telling ourselves and switch any negative thought over to a positive thought.

Studies have shown that successful people are the ones who forgive themselves quickly and move on. Michael Jordan is a perfect example. He once said, "I have failed so many times in my life, and that is why I have succeeded." So don't be so hard on yourself when you fail. Know that you are winning because you are doing it. You cannot get better at something if you're doing that thing you want to be doing.

Your Desires Are Important, but They Are Not Everything

Another critical aspect to understand is your *desires*. Every single choice we make is because we *think* it will make us feel better. However, sometimes when we get what we desire, it isn't what we need. Each desire stems from your beliefs about life. Take a minute to contemplate the things you want the most out of this life. What are your deepest heart's desires?

Many people desire the same things: a successful marriage, a shiny new car, being at the goal weight, traveling, etc. Other cravings and desires may stem from a childhood problem, lack, or trauma. If you didn't have much food growing up, you might think that there will never be enough food, so you overeat or hoard food. Or you might think that you are not loved, so you seek out attention from everybody.

Each seed of desire is in you because it's a part of your soul's evolution. It was placed there by a family member or some experience along your path that made you feel like you needed that in your life. It's time to look at all of your desires, develop a healthy understanding of why you have them, and learn how to recognize the desires that serve you and let go of the ones that do not.

I like to ask people what their heart's desire is or what legacy would they like to leave behind. Then I like to encourage them by telling them that there is no reason they can't have what they desire. Some people wonder, "Who am I to be great?", "Who am I to have people admire me?", "Who am I to be super thin and on the cover of a magazine?", or "Who am I to have a lot of money and be able to support people all across the globe?" My question is "Who are you not to be?" We are all equal, and we all have the potential to be great. There is not one person who deserves something more than another. Everybody deserves peace, happiness, and to live at the highest expression of their ultimate being.

Avoid Building a Negative Community

What drives me bonkers and why I only keep a small group of friends is because I do not like to talk about the negative news or misfortunate things going on in the world. I have an awareness of what is going on, but I choose not to dwell on the negative. I have learned that we are creatures who build a community around negativity. Why do we do this as a society? It is essential to think about the positive and *build* up the positive if we want to have a positive environment. We're going about this all wrong, and it is no wonder the world is in the state it is in; because we keep perpetuating the negative by focusing on it.

Someone might, for example, complain that "My husband didn't put the garage door down, so all the leaves blew into the garage," or "My brothers kids are so rambunctious." The problem is that they complain to the wrong person most of the time. It won't help your marriage if you complain about it to your co-workers. It won't help your brother's kids if you tell anyone other than your brother about them. All we do when we talk like this is spread negativity.

It is rare to hear people talk about the great things they have accomplished. If you speak about your triumphs and achievements, those around you may perceive what you are doing as bragging, or they may simply be jealous that you have achieved something they have not.

Instead, many groups of people commiserate around negativity. Communities built around negativity keep us stuck. They do nothing to help us evolve or change anything about the circumstances. When we constantly talk about the negative, it keeps us in that realm and energy. When we focus on the negative, we will continue to get that negativity in our life. It is not until you change your mental state and your frequency that you will attract the positive.

Become a change agent! Take a look at your life and the people you build a community of negativity with. Tell them, "I've noticed something that I'm doing, and I no longer want to do it. Please gently remind me when I begin to complain." They may not recognize it because they are not the one who initially wanted the change to begin with. This may also create a finger-pointing environment, so remember that all change is ultimately up to you.

If you find that the group of people you hang out with no longer supports your vision and goals, it may be time to find a more like-minded group of friends. It doesn't mean you have to be mean or disown those friends. You simply begin to walk down a different path. Remember that the Universe supports you. As you make this choice, the Universe will bring you that which matches your energy.

Becoming aware is the first step. The second step is to change the negative stories and begin to tell yourself new ones. The best way to make our dreams reality is to think about how the result will feel and look. Then you can consider what you have to do. Just think backward. What do you have to do to get to where you want to be? What choices would you need to make? What are the steps to get to that place?

I learned a while back that there were people I needed to disassociate myself from or simply not tell my goals to. The reason was that my experiences with them or their reactions to my goals were not experiences that would lead me down the path that I wanted to go. These people were close friends of mine, even family members. I knew that even spending time with them was not going to bring me where I wanted to end up, so I started finding new things to do that empowered me and made me feel good about myself.

To help you understand who these people may be in your life, here are a few examples: It could be the people who question you or make you feel bad for eating healthy or exercising. It could be the people who want to pull you away from the things that make you happy because having you do something for them (their goals) will make them feel happier (they are not concerned about your goals). It could be people who want to keep you from changing. Change threatens people, and often when you begin to change, they will want to pull you back to where you once were. It's like the crabs in the bucket. If one crab starts to crawl out, other crabs will grab at it and pull it back down. Eventually, the crab quits trying to crawl out.

I learned that I needed to put on a suit of armor when I was around certain people to protect my energy field. Over the years, I realized that these were often my family members. Family members have a tendency to keep you exactly where you are because your change threatens the status quo and the norm. I am not saying that most family members want to hold you back or keep you stuck. It's just what often happens if you threaten their truth (their perception of you) and their norm. Many family members are completely supportive but beware of those who seem threatened by your stepping out and wanting something better.

Let's face it, change is hard for everyone, not just you, so when you start to change from the people you are closest too, you will get reactions. Sometimes you will be met with resistance. Sometimes you will be met with love and acceptance. And sometimes you will be met with angry attempts to pull you back to where they want you.

The key to your success is knowing what you want, who you are (as an independent person), and what you need to do to keep yourself on track.

Sometimes your elevation requires your isolation until you're met with like energy in someone else. Trust me. It will happen. I pray all the time that the Universe will send me angels – people who need what I have to offer or someone who can help me with something. Helping me also helps them. Every time I have done this, the Universe delivers. I call them my Angel Team, and they know who they are.

Find a Supportive Tribe

My advice is to find a tribe that you *can* tell your truths too – people who are on the same mission as you. Hire a mentor. Find those who understand your struggles and will help lift you up when you fail instead of keeping you down. Find those who you can be real with, those who will still be there when you show your true colors.

Years ago, I paid to join a group that I knew would keep me accountable to myself and my goals. Success was only a natural byproduct of sticking to the plan. Eventually, I outgrew that group, and then I created the figureFIT! community based on the support I wanted.

It's happening all over Facebook; tribes of like-minded groups for entrepreneurs, authors, podcasters, sports enthusiasts, day-traders, and the list goes on and on.

When you find the right tribe of people, you can be vulnerable and be seen for who you are. Then you can be supported and guided toward the "you" that you want to be. You can start sharing your wins, and everyone will be happy for you because they know how hard you have worked. When you start sharing your successes with the right people, they will be there to help you and build you up. The key to your happiness and growth is finding the tribe that is going through what you are going through and can help support you.

When you receive pushback from people in your environment, you must understand that people often react because they feel bad about their choices or they are projecting on to you their own perceived inadequacies. The best response is to hold on to your truth and why you are doing what you are doing.

Here is an example: You are eating healthy food at work, and someone says, "Oh, there you go again, eating that salad. Why don't you just have a burger?" You can say, "I do have a hamburger when it's time for that." Or you could say, "This is what I choose to eat because it is the healthiest choice for me. I don't talk about the foods you bring in, so I would appreciate if you respected my choices of food." You could also say, "Yes, I'd love to eat what you're eating. That spaghetti looks awesome. But I'd pay the price later if I ate that because I've realized that I have intolerances to certain foods, and I do not eat gluten products."

It is an excellent opportunity to educate them. People think they have the right to say whatever they please about your weight and food. Personally, I think they say such things because deep down they wish they had the willpower to be doing what you are doing. They are projecting that on to you.

So remember to shine love back to others because ultimately they will respect you for what you are doing. Continue down your path and be an example. Soon those who react negatively to you will come to you and ask for help. Be the light because the world needs the light you have to give.

I'm completely in love with the figureFIT! member community. The women and men in this group are extremely supportive and forthcoming. I learn something each week from them, and I love the tremendous amount of support they give to each other. Members have made great friendships with each other. It is a great place to come together and be uplifted. I've heard first hand from many members that the group coaching calls have helped them make drastic changes in their lives. They may ask a question themselves or hear a question from another member, and each question and answer helps to support each person who reads or hears it.

One of my clients mentioned on a group coaching call that she eats when she is bored. She recognizes it when it happens, and she even has a little voice in her head saying, "You should probably stop eating these cookies." She said she is aware of it when it is happening and can't seem to stop herself. I asked her if she had begun the 21-Day Health and Wellness meditation series in the meditation library, and she said, "Not yet." I explained to her that in those moments where she is aware of what is happening yet choosing not to listen to her higher-self, she is doing something that is against her soul's (internal guide) nudging and the process of meditation will help her to begin to listen to this voice. Our soul is always going to know what is best for us, and it is always talking to us. It is when we do not listen to it that we create pain in our lives. I told my client that the problem was not the fact that she ate a cookie unless her internal guide was telling her no beforehand. But if she reached for her third or fourth cookie, and her internal guide was telling her, "Stop doing this! You don't need to do this," then she needed to change her environment immediately and go do something else.

This is where I came up with, "Stop, drop and meditate." In those moments when you find yourself doing something you no longer wish to be doing, and you get a nudge from your internal guide, you need to heed the call of the soul. You must stop what you are doing, and go meditate or go for a walk. You must leave the space you are in and go somewhere else and do something else. Go within and search yourself for why you are doing what you are doing.

In these moments, come to yourself with loving kindness and know that you are strong enough to face yourself in those moments. When you know that you are safe, supported, and *can* make changes, your life will forever be happier once you finally begin to listen to that inner guide.

CHAPTER 4
Set Yourself Up to Win

"Perception is a mirror, not a fact, and what I look at is my state of mind reflected outward."

– A Course in Miracles

We all have reasons why change happens in our lives. Usually, it boils down to three scenarios. The first common scenario is that we are sick of something, and we want it to be different. Most of the time, we want things to be different because we are tired of our current situation. This goes for many things in our lives. It might be that we are overweight, or we are sick of our jeans being too tight, or we want to look better in our swimsuit. It could be that we are tired of fighting with our boyfriend, girlfriend, or spouse, so we want out of the relationship. Or we might be sick and tired of being addicted to something, so we decide it's time to quit. Our desire for change always stems from wanting to increase our happiness.

Another reason we go through change is if something has gone wrong in our life. Though we do not necessarily want change, we need change. For example, you go through recurrent bouts of digestive problems because something you eat is not good for you. You do not want to give up the food because you like it, yet you need to give it up because it's harmful to your body.

The third reason we experience change is because it is forced upon us. A severe illness, death, losing one's job, or some traumatic event all are reasons we could be forced to make a change.

Many people do not like to make changes in their life. However, it's a necessary part of life. If you look around, you will see that everything always changes. Nothing remains the same. You fool yourself if you think that something stays the way it is. No day is exactly like the day before or the day after. But that, my friend, is a good thing. It means that change should not be looked upon as an insurmountable task or with fear, which is what many of us do.

People often think that changing things in their life is a huge undertaking, and they do not even want to begin because they don't like being uncomfortable. They feed themselves excuse after excuse as to why they are the way they are. Then they remain in the same place, doing the same things over and over again and having the same problems over and over again.

Most of the time, people don't realize that they are telling themselves excuses because they believe the stories that they tell themselves. They believe that they are sick. They believe that their condition runs in the family. They believe that they are too busy to work out. The truth is these stories are just repeated thoughts that have become habits of the mind. However, once someone makes up his or her mind to change, the decision is done. They have all the power inside of themselves to do it; they just need guidance.

Take a moment to think about your biggest dreams and desires. I know you have them. We all do. They may be buried under dust, but that does not mean that they do not exist. Close your eyes and think for a minute. What would you do or have if it could be anything? Imagine that anything is possible and nothing is holding you back. What would you do? Who would you help? What would you want your legacy to be? Go ahead; think about it.

Creating Your Vision Board

Do you have it? Okay. Now is the time to have some fun. One of the best ways to set yourself on a path to manifest your goals is to create a visual reminder of your dreams. Have you ever created a vision board? A vision board is a visual reminder of the things that you would do or have if you could have or do anything in the world. Think back to those dreams. They may be buried under dust, but they have been placed in your heart for a reason. Your dreams represent something larger: a path to freedom, happiness, peace, security, and more.

Below, write a few words that come to mind when you think about your dreams. How would living that life feel to you?

Living my dreams would make me feel:

_____

_____

_____

_____

Knowing how you want to *feel* is the best way to start manifesting the life of your desire. Everything in your life right now is a result of what you have created. Every thought, desire, belief, and action of yours has shaped your life up to now. You may have been holding on to old beliefs (limiting beliefs) that were passed on to you by your parents, family members, friends, or even teachers. But now it's time to look at your life and see if it is exactly how you want it to be. My guess is that it's not, so now is the time to throw out your old ways of thinking and build a bridge to a new mindset and a new way of life.

I believe that the Universe has our back and is always supporting what we believe is true. It's time for you to start believing that too. If you do not like certain things about your life – your body, your finances, or your love life – it's time to take a long look at your choices, past influences, and long-held belief systems. Then start to make new choices and think new thoughts that lead you down the road towards the life that you want to create. Writing down your long-held beliefs is a powerful way to see the delusion in them. As you write, you begin to see what is true and what is untrue for you. Then you can build new thoughts based on what it is you truly want. Help the Universe to support you. Find the things you love about life and show gratitude. The Universe will always give you more of what you love (or hate); it's all about your focus.

I remember a time when I very often would say, "I can't afford to do that." And you know what, I couldn't afford it, and I never would with that mindset. It wasn't until I started learning about the Law of Attraction and began to realize that my thoughts and words created everything in my life that things began to change. Instead of saying, "I can't afford," I would say, "I have everything I need to do what I need to do." Then I started seeing subtle shifts in what would come my way. As I changed my thoughts, the vibration of what I was sending out changed as well. It may sound strange, but I want you to give this new way of thinking a try.

Now that you know your dreams and what you want your legacy to be, it's time to create a visual plan to help you get there. This plan is the vision board. The vision board is a visual representation of the *feelings* that you must feel to manifest the life of your dreams. It's not just about wanting a new car, house, or a bunch of money in the bank, or giving back and helping people (and putting a photo of it on a board). It's also about creating a plan that will help you feel the feelings that will draw in that life. There is a bigger reason behind every decision you make, and that reason is usually to bring you a sense of security or comfort. Everything you do is associated with a deeper desire of how you want to feel.

Head to a store that sells poster boards and buy a thick poster board that can stand on its own. On your board, you will glue words, photos, and other inspirational items that will help you visualize your dreams every single day. When you think of the person who you long to become, you begin doing the things that will propel you towards your goals.

Find illustrations of what you need to do, ways that you want to feel, and the end goal. All of this together creates a powerful matrix for you and the Universe to draw upon. The Law of Attraction states that what we focus on, we draw into our lives.

When I wanted to write my first book, I put images of the word "write," images of my favorite books, and book signing photos, etc., on my vision board. Seeing this vision board every day propelled me to do the things that would manifest those dreams. Little by little, I started to make room for writing. It was a slow process to start, but then after about a year, it grew to an hour a day in my already packed schedule. I fell in love with what I was doing because it aligned with my larger goal.

Your vision board can be an elaborate project of images, words, and phrases that you put together on a poster board. It can also be a simple, bulleted list you make on a sheet of paper or in a Word document. It can even be as simple as a post-it note with three major goals you want to achieve that you stick on your bathroom mirror. I have done all of these, and I will say that taking a couple hours to create your board is time well spent. It can be one of the best ways to ensure that change happens and success sticks. The reason is that you will begin to do the things that you need to do unconsciously every time you see that vision board. Every day, week, and month, your brain will go to work helping you to create ways to manifest the ideas on that board. And you will be amazed at the synchronicities the Universe delivers to you.

A synchronicity is when the Universe provides the perfect person or thing at the right moment. Many angels will appear on your path. Remember to give thanks for every synchronicity you see. When you bless them and give thanks, you will receive more and more to be thankful for. When synchronicities that I knew with all of my being were from God (or the Universe) first started happening in my life, I would fall to my knees with tears of pure gratitude in my eyes. Gratitude is the key. It always brings more to be grateful for.

I created my first vision board one cold January day many years ago. I put it in my bedroom, so every time I would go in there and every time

I would go to bed, I would see it. Just by seeing my board daily, I made conscious (and unconscious) choices to do certain things that would get the balls rolling. I made phone calls, connected with people who knew more than I did, or prioritized actions that I knew I needed to take.

Seven months after I had created my first vision board, I realized that everything that I wanted was happening. I was doing all the things I needed to be doing to propel me forward. Some of the items were completed, and I was on to other significant goals. I was thrilled. As I reflected on my year, I remembered little things that had happened that helped bring my visions to fruition. I realized how the vision board had helped me make conscious choices towards the things I wanted for myself. The one major thing I learned was that I needed to dream bigger. My next board was going to have larger more elaborate goals along with small actions that led all the way up to those larger goals.

Now I make a vision board every year, sometimes every six months. I even have workshops at my yoga studio where I teach others how to create these magical boards. I have hosted get-togethers at my house with friends and family where we have created powerful architectural plans for our lives. Most of my boards, I have created when I have been by myself, but you can develop stronger relationships with friends and family members by doing it together with them.

It is easy to sit back and let time pass while saying, "I'll do it next week" or "I have plenty of time to _____ (fill in the blank)." But the truth is, we do not have all the time in the world. *Time waits for no one*, and if you do not take action, then another day goes by while your dreams patiently wait for you to answer the call.

Dream with me and do not underestimate the power of the process. Entrepreneurs, authors, athletes, and millionaires across the globe use it. It is how you can tell the Universe exactly what you're willing to do to help manifest your dreams.

Visualization

The next step is visualization. It might be the most important step of all.

When I was in high school, I was on the pompon squad (dance team). We would go to summer camp every year at Indiana University. While we were there, we would usually learn two to three new dances each day and a total of about seven per week. At the end of the week, we would have to perform all the dances in front of the judges and all of the other girls who were at the camp.

I was always afraid of not being able to learn the routines because dancing did not come naturally to me. We only got one chance to learn the dance and ask the instructor questions about technique. The next day, we would move on to another dance routine. One of the stories I told myself was that since I had not grown up in dance classes like many of the other girls on my team, and since I had just started dancing when I was a freshman, I would not be as good as them. The others learned the routines on the first day, but I struggled getting a grasp on them. I mostly stood watching the others, or I was one or two steps behind.

One of the instructors (an angel) saw me struggling during the practice. She told me, "Tonight when you're lying in bed, I want you to run through the dance in your head and visualize yourself doing the steps with grace and precise techniques. Imagine yourself nailing the routine!"

Every night at pompon camp, we would play, talk, tease the younger girls, dance around in lingerie (*trying* to feel sexy), and put on comedic skits for each other. We had a lot of fun. It was surprising that anyone danced well because we didn't get much sleep, and we eat crappy food!

That night, I almost forgot the advice the instructor had given me. But when I lay in bed and fear about the next day set in, I remembered the angel's directions to visualize the routine. "Ok, here it goes," I thought. That night, I ran through each routine once. I fell asleep as I was trying to run through them once more.

The next morning, I remember waking up and feeling like my efforts were not good enough because I didn't feel that I had spent enough time on it. But this was the moment of truth. Once we got into our groups for the morning, we would run through the dance routines from the previous day, with the music, and without stopping.

I was in complete shock. I danced the dance, and I was in sync with the music. At that moment, I knew the visualization was magic. Sure, there were moves that needed perfecting, but the fact that I had learned the routines was huge. Going from watching the squad's best dancers to doing the routine with them was a great feeling.

The visualizing technique paid off. I went on to earn a blue ribbon (first place) in every routine that I performed. In addition to the blue ribbons, I was selected to audition for the All-American Dance Team, which I did and made with only a handful of others. Believing in yourself and pursuing your dreams is powerful. Visualization is a powerful tool that helped me to become one of the best dancers on the pompon squad.

When I competed in fitness, I visualized myself walking on stage. I actually did the walk. I practiced the walk and my turn, and I imagined how it would sound and feel. I used all of my senses to give my body the experience of doing this successfully.

Let's dip our toes in this together and give it a try. Take two minutes right now to do this small but very powerful exercise: Close your eyes and start to bring forth images in your mind of what your biggest dream will feel like. How does it look? Who is there? How does it feel? What can you feel happening in your body? How does it sound? What are people saying to you, and what are you saying to those around you? What are you saying to yourself? Allow the feelings that this experience would give you come up now. Take them all in and dream big for a moment.

If you feel like your mind is blocked, take a deep breath and keep your eye on the goal. Let your heart's desire swell in you. Let yourself think beautiful thoughts about what you want to achieve. What kind of financial success will this bring you? How will you help others with this financial success? Where will this lead you in your life, and what will you begin to create next? Let the desire build up in you. If you can imagine it, you can have it.

Athletes, chess players, entrepreneurs, and motivational speakers all visualize their goals and dreams. Research has shown that our brain can't tell the difference between visualized images and reality.

We have both a conscious and a subconscious mind. The conscious mind is what we choose to think about at that moment, and we can only focus on one thing at a time. The subconscious works slightly differently than the conscious, and it's very powerful. The subconscious mind sees a complete picture of everything that is happening all at once. It is constantly aware of the input from all of your senses, and it helps the body assemble all it needs for that moment.

Your conscious mind is fantastic at coming up with ideas, yet it is easily distracted, so attaining goals is something your subconscious does. The subconscious mind can remember billions of things in perfect sequence, not only for minutes at a time but also for your lifetime.

I teach my clients that the power is in the present moment because that is where life happens. However, there is immense power in your subconscious brain. When you envision a story, your subconscious will watch it play out and think it is real. "The subconscious mind is a captive audience for the movies we play in our head,"[6] and it believes they are true.

Think about a time when you got worked up about a story you were telling yourself. It was not even happening, yet the mere thought of it caused measurable biological changes. Your pulse raced, your breath quickened, and you may have even acted upon this story in your head, only later to realize that you overreacted.

---

6 Understand Your Brain to Use Visualization - johnassaraf. com. (2010, November 26). Retrieved August 13, 2015, from http:// johnassaraf. com/law-of-attraction/understand-your-brain-to-use-visualization

When we make up stories about ourselves, our life, or situations we are in, and we play them in our mind, our body can't tell them apart from real events. That is why it is imperative to visualize what we want. This visualization will begin to reshape your perception of reality, and once that happens, reality conforms to that perception. Your life script visualized and acted upon can change the course of your life.

Five Steps of the Visualization Process

Begin by visualizing your dreams. Involve all your senses: touch, sound, sight, and even smell and taste. Engage your emotions: laugh, smell, and celebrate the victory. You may feel weird when you do this, but remember that you are calling in your biggest dreams and desires. If it makes you feel better, be by yourself when you do this visualization exercise.

Then take on different perspectives. See yourself accomplishing your goals and things coming to fruition. If you want to win an award, imagine yourself on stage being handed that award. If you long for a promotion, imagine the conversation with your boss, the praise, and the feeling that the raise will bring. No matter what, when you begin to align your-self with the energy of the positive feelings you wish to have, you will start to call in other energies of the same frequency. Then take a step further and visualize yourself in the second person seeing you receiving this award. Then imagine taking in the situation from the third person, being in the crowd and seeing you succeeding.

The third step is beginning to live as if you have succeeded in your goal. Begin to dress and talk accordingly. What will happen is you will begin to look and act like the person you want to be. The mind is very powerful. What you think you are, you are. If you think you are overweight, lazy and ugly, then you are. If you think you are beautiful and sexy, then you will manifest those energies.

The fourth step is combining visualization with affirmative self-talk. Say what you would like to be said in the first, second, and third person as if you have already achieved your goal. More to do with affirmations is coming in the following chapter.

Last but not least, create that vision board. Keep it in a place where you can see it daily. Make a brand new vision board for your dreams and goals every year.

Set Yourself Up to Win

Now that you have a vision of what you want your life to look and feel like, it's time to create a plan.

My mottos for my figureFIT! members are, "Baby steps to change," and "Make the best choice in every moment; only focusing on what you can do right here and now." Focusing on the big picture tends to overwhelm us. Instead, focus on baby steps and making the best choice each moment.

When we have a goal in sight, we are more likely to take actions towards it. When I am not working towards a goal, I often feel like a fish out of water, flopping around, because I do not know in which direction I am going.

It is now time to create goals regarding your big dreams. Break down your dreams into small actions that you can take monthly, weekly, and daily.

Get a journal that you can write in every night, documenting your wins and failures. Set up reminders on your phone for the daily tasks that you will need to do to keep you on target. Take your "before photo." Know your macros. Your macros are the number of protein, fat, and carbohydrates you need to consume every day based on your height, weight, and age. If you need help figuring that out, head over to figurefitlife.com/shop and let us find it out for you by purchasing the product called "Calculate My Macros."

Find an accountability partner. On the figureFIT! Lifestyle Program, there is a whole community supporting each other. Come to figurefitlife. com and join this community. Every Sunday, we plan our week ahead. We schedule when we will work out and what we will eat. This way, we set ourselves up to *win*.

Only buy the food that you plan to eat that week. Throw out any goodies left over from the weekend or festivities so that those do not make their way into your week.

Use figureFIT! Worksheet II: "Set Yourself Up to Win," which you will find in the Appendix, to prepare yourself for negative scenarios by planning and visualizing.

Where are you likely to fail if you do not have a plan? Where we fail is just a red flag of an area that needs special attention. We can hardwire new habits and shatter limiting beliefs by being aware of what throws us off and what limiting stories we tell ourselves.

Set up affirmations: positive statements of what is going well and what you do want. Place them strategically. For example, I put affirmations on my phone in the morning when I wake up to start my day off right, mid-day, and in the evenings. Prior to my self-awareness practice, I would mindlessly find myself in the kitchen looking for something to eat when I wasn't even hungry. My strategically placed affirmations helped me to stay strong on my journey towards great health and a fit body. For ideas of affirmations you can use, turn to the "figureFIT! Affirmations" in the Appendix.

If you can envision it and dream it, you can surely have it. Our desires and our dreams are placed in our hearts for a reason, and it's time to start taking steps towards manifesting those dreams and goals.

CHAPTER 5
The Good and Bad of Stress

Happiness is our only job.

– Liz Nierzwicki

From shingles to depression to sleepless nights, stress has affected me in a big way over the years. It has forced me to find ways to cope that were healthy. I became a yoga teacher solely because of the stress relief I felt after a class one day. I knew that I needed it in my life on a daily basis because of the lifestyle I lived. I am a go-getter, and I chase my dreams. I'm the first to say that I am addicted to creating businesses, books, and other tools that help people. Often, I don't sit down to rest until I'm forced to. This way of living didn't support me for very long, which you'll learn more about that in this chapter.

I know I'm not alone in experiencing stress. Our society is very driven and with so many things vying for our attention, it is often hard to get the rest and rejuvenation we need. Constantly being on the go and chronic stress can affect your health without you even realizing it. It can manifest itself in the body in many ways. If you're sick, you might think genes or bacteria is to blame, but it could very well be stress from your life manifesting itself in your body. Chronic stress can have detrimental effects on the body and can be the culprit for many diseases and other health related problems. But it can also be helpful.

Neuroscientist and heart researchers have determined that it is how you view stress that ultimately matters.

In the first part of this chapter, I'm going to dive into some recent studies that have been conducted on humans and mice that were undergoing stress or were put under stress to test its effects. In the later part of this chapter, we will cover how stress is beneficial and can actually help you.

Effects of Stress

Research has confirmed (and you may already be familiar with) that stress can cause the following:

- Headaches

- Muscle tension or pain

- Knots in our upper back, neck, and hips

- Chest pains

- Fatigue

- Chronic tiredness

- Change in your sex drive

- Upset stomach, diarrhea or constipation

- Insomnia and other sleep problems

- Rapid breathing

When it comes to our mood, stress can cause anxiety, restlessness, lack of motivation, lack of focus, irritability or anger, and sadness or depression. Common effects of stress on your behavior can include overeating, undereating, outbursts of anger, drug or alcohol abuse, tobacco abuse, and social withdrawal.

We all know that chronic stress is not a good thing. When you are in tune with your body with the help of a self-awareness practice such as yoga or mindfulness, you might feel when stress comes on. But if you do not know when you are stressed, if you always feel like you are under pressure, overwhelmed, anxious, or frazzled, the effects can add up to something quite dangerous.

A recent animal study conducted by Wake Forest University researchers showed that stress could help cancer cells survive against anti-cancer drugs. The study, published in the Journal of Clinical Investigation, was done on mice induced to experience stress by being exposed to the scent of a predator. When experiencing this stress, an anti-cancer drug administered to the mice was less effective at killing cancer cells, and the cancer cells were actually *kept* from dying.[7]

In another study from Yale University, researchers suggest that stressful events, like going through a divorce or being laid off, can shrink your brain.[7] We learned earlier that when we are "asleep" in the evaluating mind, the brain is in automatic mode, and it is not utilizing the part of the brain that keep the mind in the present moment. When we are in this other mode of mind chronically, it is no wonder why the gray matter in the experiencing mind would shrink.

According to research in the Journal of Molecular Psychiatry, stress can prematurely age kids. "The extreme duress that a child experiences when exposed to violence early on could lead to premature aging of his or her cells."[7] This study followed 236 children born in England and Wales between the ages of 5 and 10.[5] This data showed that those who had been bullied, witnessed violent acts, or were victims of violence, those children had shorter telomeres than other children.

---

[7] Chan, A. (2013, February 4). Stress Health Effects: 10 Scary Things It's Doing To Your Body. Retrieved August 12, 2015, from http://www.huffingtonpost.com/2013/02/04/stress-health-effects-cancer-immune-system_n_2599551.html

Telomeres are the protective caps on the ends of chromosomes that affect how quickly cells age. When your telomeres disintegrate, you age faster. There are combinations of DNA and protein that protect the ends of chromosomes and help them remain stable. As the telomeres become shorter, and their structural integrity weakens, the cells age and die off more quickly.

In recent years, many studies have been done on telomeres. They have become associated with a broad range of aging-related diseases including cancer, stroke, vascular dementia, heart problems, obesity, osteoporosis, and diabetes. A small UCSF pilot study is the first study that shows that changes in diet, exercise, stress management, and social support can result in longer telomeres.

Dr. Dean Ornish, UCSF clinical professor of medicine, and founder and president of the Preventive Medicine Research Institute, has determined through his extensive amounts of research that

> Our genes, and our telomeres, are not necessarily our fate. So often people think 'Oh, I have bad genes, there's nothing I can do about it. But these findings indicate that telomeres may lengthen to the degree that people change how they live. Research indicates that longer telomeres are associated with fewer illnesses and longer life.[8]

Knowing that we can actually change our genetic expression through lifestyle is a major win in science. I've often heard, "there's nothing I can do about it, my whole family is this way." I personally never bought into that logic. I have always believed that we have much power over our life and health. It is what we choose to focus on and do that matters. If we think, "Oh well, my whole family is fat, so what's the point, I'm going to be fat too," and then don't put in our best effort to be healthy and create a new trajectory, we will be fat just like them. It's a no-brainer.

---

[8] Fernandez, E. (2013, September 16). Lifestyle Changes May Lengthen Telomeres, A Measure of Cell Aging. Retrieved August 12, 2015, from https://www.ucsf.edu/news/2013/09/108886/lifestyle-changes-may-lengthen-telomeres-measure-cell-aging

Stress can also affect your offspring's genes:

The effects of stress on a person's genes may be passed on from generation to generation, according to a recent Science study — suggesting stress's effects may not just take a toll on the person itself, but the person's progeny, too. New Scientist reported on the research, which was conducted in mouse germ cells (before they become eggs or sperm) by University of Cambridge researchers. They reported that certain markings to the genes, influenced by outside factors like stress, are generally thought to be erased in the next generation. But the new study shows that some of these markings to the genes still exist in the next generation.[9]

Stress can spur on depressive symptoms:

Researchers at the U.S. National Institute on Mental Health conducted several experiments on mice, where they noted how stress affected their behavior. They found that stress was linked with depression-like behaviors, such as giving up swimming in a plastic cylinder and lengthening the response time it took to eat food. "I think the findings fit well with the idea that stress can cause depression or that stressful situations can precipitate depression".[9]

Are you stressed out reading this? Well take a deep breath in and then exhale out, just a few more research findings to go.

Stress increases the risk of chronic diseases.

It's not just the stress, but how you react to it, that could have an impact on your health down the road, according to a new study from Pennsylvania State University researchers. Published in the journal

[9] Chan, A. (2013, February 4). Stress Health Effects: 10 Scary Things It's Doing To Your Body. Retrieved August 12, 2015, from http://www.huffingtonpost.com/2013/02/04/stress-health-effects-cancer-immune-system_n_2599551.html

Annals of Behavioral Medicine, the study found that people who were more stressed out and anxious about the stresses of everyday life were, in turn, more likely to have chronic health conditions (such as heart problems or arthritis) 10 years later, compared with people who viewed things through a more relaxed lens.

Stress also raises the risk of stroke.

Stressed-out people may have a higher stroke risk than their more mellowed-out peers, according to an observational study published in the Journal of Neurology, Neurosurgery and Psychiatry. "Compared with healthy age-matched individuals, stressful habits and type A behavior are associated with high risk of stroke.

Stress does a number on your heart, and it increases the risk of heart attack.

Feeling anxious and stressed is linked with a 27 percent higher risk of heart attack — the same effect smoking five cigarettes a day has on the heart. "These findings are significant because they are applicable to nearly everyone". Reuters reported on another study, conducted by researchers at St. Luke's Mid America Heart Institute, that showed that stress is linked with a 42 percent higher risk of dying in the two years after being hospitalized for a heart attack.

When Stress Is Actually Good for You

Stress is inevitable. Every single one of us is bound to endure stress, but what is important is to build stress-balancing opportunities into our daily lives. My protocol around stress is to put into practice *daily* tools that help to relieve stress such as workouts, reading, meditation, yoga, spending time outdoors, or anything that naturally calms me.

I was working with a private client and after a private yoga session, I asked him how he was feeling. He said, "It's amazing that I have gone for weeks, even months, so wound up, not taking the time to de-stress. Going from day to day like this is awful, and it's no wonder my body is so tight in certain areas."

This fast-paced world we live in is great when we know how to balance it. But most people, if they're like my client, going from day to day layering stress on top of stress, will be sorry in the long run if they do not put tools into place daily to help them balance out the stress. In today's society, it's more important than ever to remember that your physical and mental health must be put at the forefront of your life.

Since stress is inevitable, it's important to view stress as helpful rather than detrimental. Here are a few ways stress is helpful:

1. Stress helps to boost brainpower by stimulating the production of brain chemicals that strengthen the connections between the neurons in the brain.

2. Stress can increase immunity in the short term by producing extra chemicals that regulate the immune system by preparing for possible injury or infection.

3. Short-term stress can make you more resilient to future stressful occurrence.

4. Stress motivates you to succeed.

5. Mild to moderate stress in pregnant moms produces offspring who show greater motor and development skills.[10]

In a recent Ted talk, the psychologist Kelly McGonigal urges us to see stress as a positive.[11] She says that stress activates the fight or flight response in the body. When this response is activated, the heart pumps

---

[10] MacMillan, A. (2014, August 18). 5 Weird Ways Stress Can Actually Be Good for You. Retrieved August 12, 2015, from http:// news. health.com/2014/08/18/5-weird-ways-stress-can-actually-be-good-for-you/

[11] How to make stress your friend. (n.d.). Retrieved August 12, 2015, from http://www.ted.com/talks/kelly_mcgonigal_how_to_make_stress_your_friend?language=en

large loads of dopamine. Most people know dopamine as the love hormone. What McGonigal mentions is that the body has a built-in mechanism to deal with stress, and that mechanism is urging us to reach out to others for support.

In 2009, I had a very stressful job, and a lot was going on in my personal life as well. All of a sudden, I started having agonizing pain in the upper right-hand part of my head where my temple is. I called my doctor and told him what was going on.

"It sounds like you have shingles," he said.

"Shingles? What the heck? Isn't that for old people?" I answered in surprise.

"Actually no," he replied. "Anybody can get shingles."

He wanted me to come to his office for a talk, so I did. He asked me questions and touched the area, and he asked me to describe the symptoms. Then he confirmed that I did indeed have shingles. He put me on a heavy dose of medication to reduce the inflammation and told me it was time to add more to my anti-stress routine.

Shingles is an inflammation of the ending of the nerves in your body, which causes them to flare up. It can be a crippling and almost debilitating pain. Even the wind blowing on my face hurt me. Once the shingles goes away, or if you have not yet had shingles, you can get the shingles vaccination. The vaccination does not guarantee that the shingles will never come back, but if it comes back, it is usually less severe. Once I was free and clear of the active shingles virus, I got it because I never wanted to experience that pain again. It's a pain I would never wish on anyone.

The doctor ordered me to do more to relax. He said, "I know you like to work out, and you practice yoga, but that doesn't seem to be enough for you. You need to incorporate other techniques to reduce stress." He told me to continue exercising, do more yoga, meditate, practice deep breathing exercises, go for walks in nature, and have orgasms daily.

"But Doc, I'm not dating anyone," I replied to his last piece of advice.

"Well, I'm sure you know how to take care of that yourself," he answered.

"Are you giving me a prescription to masturbate?" I asked.

"Do you need a prescription for that?" He asked.

I told him that I had always felt a little guilty about masturbation. He looked at me a bit funny and said that it was a very good and natural way for the body to release tension. Due to the tension I was under, he recommended me to have an orgasm every day, and he said that there was nothing to feel guilty about.

I tell you this story because over the years, as I have helped women with their stress levels and asked them this question, I've found that many feel guilty about it. Some believe it would be frowned upon by their religion. Others feel guilty if and when they do it. As a result, they do not do it. Knowing what I know about the body and fully accepting masturbation as an acceptable form of stress relief, I have embraced it, and I recommend it to my clients as well. If you need permission, here I give it to you: It's okay to masturbate. You do not *need* anyone else to take care of you. In fact, it's important that you know your body and can take care of yourself when you feel the need. Those who work at home can easily take a time-out when stress comes on. Those who work in the corporate world will just have to take care of themselves at the end of the day. There would be many fewer unplanned babies, affairs, and STDs if we all were taught to self-soothe in this way. In fact, there would probably be a lot less war and fighting.

Since stress management is so important to a healthy body and mind, I have incorporated techniques for it in the figureFIT! Lifestyle Program. I encourage our members to use the yoga videos, deep breathing exercises, and meditations in the meditation library to de-stress every day. These techniques will help. Workouts and anything else you can do that is healthy will help as well. Turning to alcohol is not a healthy option, so focus on the list below and start to find your stress relief tools.

Rest and Rejuvenation

Life will always call us to do what must be done. But when you hurry through life without a break to connect back to your spirit daily and find the peace within, it will leave you feeling disconnected and frazzled. It will cause frustration in all aspects of your life. Be careful not to let endless tasks take you away from your true self.

It's time to relax and take pleasure in life. You may have a busy lifestyle, kids, a business, multiple jobs, etc., but you must take time every day to connect back to the spirit that lives within. Peace lies within you, and all you have to do is sit in silence for about 10 to 15 minutes per day to allow yourself to sit in the stillness that is you. When you allow yourself this time, you tap into the wisdom and peace that is always vibrating there.

Make it a priority to engage in peaceful thinking and finding small segments of time throughout your day to enjoy the beauty of life that surrounds you. In those moments, let your heart and mind be filled with all the things that you are thankful for. Let only these thoughts permeate your mind and notice the feeling of peace wash over you. Your connection to your spirit will bring you great assistance and clarity, but it can only be achieved through regular relaxation and meditation. By implementing periods of rest throughout your day, you will find that this is far more productive for you than unceasing action.

Stress Management Tools

If you have stress symptoms, start by taking small steps throughout your day to manage your stress. You will have numerous health benefits, and you can use the effects of stress to your benefit. Here are some stress management strategies that I encourage my clients to practice:

- Physical activity

- Relaxation techniques such as breathing exercises

- Meditation

- Yoga

- Being in nature

- Plenty of sleep

- A well-balanced diet

- Avoiding alcohol

- Avoiding caffeine

- Avoiding smoking

- Avoiding negative or stressful people

- Having an orgasm daily

We live in a fast-paced world with a lot of people and companies vying to get your attention. For that reason, it's important to take the time to slow down every day and reconnect with your soul. When you notice yourself feeling anxious, stressed, depressed, angry, or anything other than joyful, take time to relax in a quiet place. Do it even if it means locking yourself in a bathroom to get away from everyone. You are worth it.

CHAPTER 6
Sleep

By now, we have all heard how important sleep is. Many don't have any issues with sleep, but life is funny; what has been a non-issue can sometimes make itself an issue based on our situations in life. Remember the stress we spoke about in the last chapter? Well, that alone can make someone an insomniac.

There are many levels of sleep issues or deprivation. Sleeping too little, sleeping too much, broken sleep, waking up multiple times in the middle of the night, snoring, and sleep apnea are just a few examples. Insomnia, not being able to fall asleep despite how tired you are, is another example. Mental issues or stress can make it more difficult for you to fall asleep as well.

There were a couple periods in my life where I went through sleepless nights. The first was when my son was a newborn. The second was when I simply had too much going on in my life, and I was struggling financially. I was a single mother, and I had a home and all that entails. The job I had was not bringing in enough money to cover all my expenses. So at night, I would contemplate ways to bring in extra money or save money – what to cut out from my life. I went from being someone who slept like a rock every night to someone who could not sleep anymore. I would lie down, my brain would start up, and then I would lie there trying to fall asleep for hours. Or if I would wake up, going back to sleep was not very likely.

The phase when my son was a newborn was a time of great beauty and love. At the same time, it was one of the hardest experiences I had gone through. My son did not sleep through the night for the first two years of his life. As a single working mother, this was like hell on earth after a while because I was exhausted. I started to understand how keeping people awake is a form of torture.

I think I aged five years during that time. It was not fun. The only thing that kept me sane was my spiritual practice and my son's adorable big eyes that stared at me while I held him. I was his rock. I was his lifeline. He needed me, and I was there for him. Luckily during that first year, I lived with my mom. When I got to my whit's end, I would wake her and ask her to help me with him so that I could sleep. I didn't like to do that often because we both worked, and we both needed sleep. I didn't want to make it her problem that I chose to be a single mother – because it was my choice. It was my struggle to deal with. I was blessed to receive her help.

I knew that this was a time in my life that would pass, but it was not without a struggle. As I said, it was two years of sleep deprivation. My mind was not in a healthy place. A couple of times during those two years, I just wanted it all to end, and I would think about not wanting to be alive anymore. Life was extremely hard, and I wondered how I was going to be able to do it. I would sit and think about all that I had to do the next day and how I was going to get through it. I knew and felt that a child is a gift from God, but all I wanted at that point was to sleep so that I could enjoy that time of his life.

The sleep deprivation I experienced during the first two years of my son's life changed me. I am a very optimistic person and always see the bright side, but this opened me up to see the dark side. I became more cynical and no longer viewed parenthood as a beautiful gift. I was in a very bleak place, and all I wanted was for my son to sleep. I vowed never to have another child. I felt I couldn't possibly do it again. Even if I were to have a helper the next time I had a child, I didn't know if I could manage.

I knew I needed to reach out for help, and I did. I reached out to my mom, sister, and aunt, and I asked them to help me with my son. I needed time away. I needed naps. I just needed a break. As time passed, and he started to sleep longer periods of time, my mindset got better, and I started to feel more normal. I started to enjoy motherhood.

As I got older, I realized that everything has an opposite. Good has a bad. Light has darkness. I had to sit with my suffering and look at it to learn what got me there so that I could avoid putting myself in that position again. I prayed a lot. I went to church, and I asked for tips on life from people who were older than me. I had to do a lot of mental work, and I stayed close to my family and the people who loved me.

Studies have shown that sleep problems may raise the risk and even directly contribute to the development of psychiatric disorders in both adults and children. I felt that when I was sleepless. I knew that my mind wasn't right. I also knew that I needed to reach out for help to keep any level of sanity that I had. I knew my baby would grow out of this phase where I got no sleep, but while it was happening, it was awful.

> The brain basis of a mutual relationship between sleep and mental health is not yet completely understood. But neuroimaging and neurochemistry studies suggest that a good night's sleep helps foster both mental and emotional resilience while chronic sleep disruption sets the stage for negative thinking and emotional vulnerability.[12]

No doubt I was struggling with certain areas in my life then. It was the hardest part of my journey. No sleep, working full time, cooking, cleaning, and playing with my son – it was all challenging.

Single mothers need help, but many don't like to ask for it. The world needs many angels. If you're a neighbor, friend, or co-worker of a single mother, ask her how you can help her. Tell her you're willing to take a sleepless night so she can have a full night. Shovel her driveway.

---

[12] Sleep and mental health - Harvard Health. (2009, July 1). Retrieved August 15, 2015, from http://www.health.harvard.edu/newsletter_article/Sleep-and-mental-health

Come over and let her take a nap while you watch the baby. Your acts of service could save someone's mental state and possibly their life. It is not an understatement.

This hardship that I went through is a large part of what has made me who I am today. It has helped shape what I want and what I do not want for my future. I have realized that sleep is one of the most important things in my life for my mental health, my son's upbringing, and my professional career.

Once my son finally started sleeping through the night at age 2, I began sleeping more as well. I began to transition out of that phase of my life, and I knew I never wanted to return. I slowly regained my physical and mental health.

As a result of these two years, I have become a self-proclaimed sleep snob. When anything gets in the way of my seven to eight hours of sleep, I immediately take action to fix it.

"Is Sleep Your Secret Weapon?" I had a client ask me this once. After thinking about it, I thought, "Yes, I think it definitely helps. So many great things are happening when the body is asleep!"

Getting good quality sleep is one of my highest priorities. Most adults should aim for at least seven to nine hours of good (solid) sleep every night. If I have less than eight hours, I'm not operating at my optimal levels, and I can tell.

What Happens When We Sleep?

Your night is composed of two parts: NREM (Non-Rapid Eye Movement) sleep, which makes up ¾ of your sleep period; and REM (Rapid Eye Movement) sleep, which occurs in the last ¼ of sleep.

NREM Stages One and Two: You drift between waking and sleeping as you disengage from your surroundings. Your heart rate evens out to a steady, slow beat, and your body temperature drops.

NREM Stages Three and Four: This is the deepest, most restorative sleep. Your heart rate is very low, and blood moves to your muscles – repairing and growing new tissue [that you worked in the day's prior figureFIT! workout.] Hormones are released that are essential to muscle growth, as well as mood and appetite regulation.

REM Stage 5: Your muscles turn off and energy is supplied to your body and brain—this is like recharging your batteries. It provides the focus and energy you need for the following day… and this is also the time when you dream.

REM sleep occurs about 90 minutes after you fall asleep, and then cycles back every 90 minutes or so throughout the night—with longer periods of REM sleep as the cycle progresses.[13]

---

[13] James, A. (2015, May 12). How to Balance Your Hormones and Burn Fat with a Good Night's Sleep. Retrieved August 12, 2015, from http://fatburningman.com/how-to-balance-your-hormones-and-burn-fat-with-a-good-nights-sleep/

During the two phases of sleep:

NREM	REM
Person is easily woken	Person is usually difficult to wake
Breathing deepens	80 percent of dreaming occurs in REM
Decrease in heart rate and blood pressure	Increase in heart rate and blood pressure
Overall decrease in body temperature	Breathing patterns vary
Decrease in muscular activity	Overall increase in body temperature
Growth hormone rises and peaks	Cortisol levels stabilize and rise towards morning
Cortisol levels fall	Peak prolactin release
Reduction in thyroid output	Increase thyroid output (metabolic rate)
	Testosterone levels increase rapidly

What Happens When You Do Not Get Enough Sleep?

I spent a good two years of my life getting an average of two to six hours of interrupted sleep per night. I would get a total of approximately six hours of broken sleep, and I always felt like crap the next day. I would be quick to anger and craving sweets. I couldn't lose weight, and I always felt like I was on the verge of a breakdown on top of numerous other health problems.

Many people in our society like to wear their lack of sleep as a badge of honor. "I'll sleep when I'm dead." Well, to be frank, they may just be dead sooner than their peers who get more sleep. In our society, overtime and 60-hour workweeks are spoken about as if they are a must to achieve great success. Many of us jump on this train and think that we need to do this to be successful. As it turns out, skipping sleep won't get us ahead. It will just make us sick. We'll get depressed, and then we'll take pills. It will also make us fat and accelerate our aging.

A recent study of 61 adults uncovered that interrupted sleep was just as bad as getting only four hours of sleep. They found the subjects were cranky, tired, craved sweets, often depressed, and had less excitement for the day. These were the results after just one night of poor sleep. Imagine the consequences of multiple nights or years of insufficient sleep.

Sleep deprivation is a big contributor to fat gain. When your natural circadian rhythms are disrupted, your body's hormones (cortisol, testosterone, and human growth hormone) are highly disrupted. Anyone who has had hormone problems will tell you that it is not something you want as it can cause major problems in the body. Here is what happens to our hormones when we do not get enough sleep.

Cortisol – When we do not get enough sleep, cortisol is the hormone that is the most affected. If it is not taken care of, it can wreak havoc on your body. When this hormone is out of whack, it can cause poor decision-making, increased blood pressure, insulin resistance, disrupted glucose management, deposits of fat in muscle tissues, and increased muscular breakdown.

When the body's glucose management is impaired, it can make you more likely to develop diabetes and cardiovascular diseases. "In fact, studies have shown that subjects who slept less than five to six hours per night were twice as likely to develop diabetes."

Normally, cortisol levels drastically decrease at your "regular" bed time, and then slowly increase throughout the sleep cycle so that you wake in the morning feeling energized. However, when you undergo just short of a week's sleep deprivation, cortisol levels have a hard time coming down at bed time.

Testosterone – the testosterone release precedes the REM stage of sleep. So it's been shown that a loss of REM sleep affects neurogenesis (growth of nervous tissue) and memory consolidation. Poor sleep affects the memory, and cognitive impairment is apparent.

Growth Hormone (GH) – "The altered rate of GH secretion during periods of sleep deprivation also has an adverse effect on insulin resistance and glucose tolerance."

Leptin – Sleep deprivation lowers leptin, an appetite-suppressing hormone released by fat cells as a signal to the brain that you are full.

Recent studies on humans reflect what we already knew about animals – those who are sleep deprived are unable to effectively regulate the release of this hormone, which simulates a state of famine accompanied by a marked increase in appetite.

Ghrelin – "Ghrelin is like the opposite of leptin – it's the appetite stimulant … and (surprise!) ghrelin levels jump up when you're sleep-deprived."

When we are not getting enough sleep, our hormones are severely affected, and it doesn't take much time before things start to get out of whack. So, let's see – your glucose tolerance is impaired, you are hungrier, *and* you are reaching for all the wrong things to eat. Fantastic!

Men and women are both affected by sleep deprivation. Men will experience poor sexual function, depression, and intensified muscle atrophy. Women are likely to experience severe depression, weight gain, as well as other mental health problems.

Sleep Better and Longer

What can we do? Make sleep a priority for your life. Here are a few ways to put sleep at the top of your list and to also make sure that it is good-quality sleep:

- Make sleep a priority in your life. The phrase, "I'll sleep when I'm dead," is spoken by people who are ignorant to just how important sleep truly is. Again, they may just be dead sooner than those who make sleep a priority.

- Take inventory of what is causing you sleep deprivation. Get rid of the unnecessary distractions and things that are not critical to your life.

- Take a yoga class after work to help you release the stress from the day and calm your central nervous system.

- Take breaks throughout the day to sit with your breath, tune in to your inner spirit, and be present in the moment.

- Get some sunshine when you wake up in the morning or early in the day—this will help reset your circadian rhythm, your body's hormone-production clock.

- Feast after sunset to kick in the "rest and digest" mode and slow cortisol production. Keep carbohydrates out of the first part of your day. Enjoy the majority before and after your workout or later in the day. Have you ever felt that relaxed feeling from a higher carbohydrate meal at night? The surge in serotonin will help you relax, and if you train after work, those additional carbohydrates will be perfect for recovery.

- Avoid caffeine after noon. "Caffeinated beverages such as coffee will stimulate the central nervous system for up to 12 hours after ingestion." Instead, reach for water to help keep you hydrated. If you work out later in the day, opt for a non-caffeinated pre-training supplement or herbal tea (e.g. Rooibos tea).

- Try to establish a sleep schedule with time built in to decompress and wind down your active mind at the end of the day. Don't read on your phone or watch TV right before falling asleep.

In fact, you should turn off your phone and any technology about an hour or two before you go to bed. Avoid electronics (including television and computers) for a couple hours before hitting the sack, and keep them out of your bedroom if possible. If you must be in front of a screen, try blue-blocking optics like Gunnar glasses.

- Drink no alcohol past 4:00 PM – Studies show that having alcohol close to bedtime may put you to sleep faster but gives you interrupted sleep throughout the night. Opt for alcohol-free beverages in the evening or if you decide to indulge, make sure that you enjoy it immediately after work. That way you can ensure that you will get to bed and have a restful slumber.

- Keep your bedroom cool and dark to help you slip into deeper sleep faster.

- I love having a fan on at night for ambient noise. A fan will help to minimize outside noises especially if you have others living in your house with you or you live near a train or noisy area.

- Don't set an alarm for snoozing. Let yourself sleep all the way up to your wake time and then if need be, snooze for one round. Why cut into perfectly good sleep time by adding broken sleep to your morning? You need that sleep, so take every second you can get.

- If you still have trouble clearing your mind at night, try yoga nidra. It's a deep relaxation practice that will help you to turn your awareness to your body and shut down the mind. In the figureFIT! meditation library, you can listen to a guided yoga nidra practice. It will shut off when complete, so if you fall asleep, you can rest assured that your meditation did too.

- Experiment with melatonin. Start with 1 to 3 mg about an hour or two before bed. If you don't notice any effect, be sure to take it before your nightly meal. Just know this, you will be ready for bed after your meal, so plan your evening accordingly.

- It is a fact that sleep deprivation does cause you to eat more during the day after–up to 22% more to be exact. For the average person, that's an extra 550 calories a day! Do that enough times in the week and you'll be wondering where all that extra weight is coming from.

- Stop your intake of water about two hours before bedtime to avoid the middle of the night bathroom run.

- The classic combination of zinc, magnesium and vitamin B6 is often used to help promote sleep with good reason. Magnesium deficiency results in lowered melatonin secretion and higher cortisol levels as well as muscle cramping and constipation: whilst Zinc is needed in the biochemical pathway to secrete melatonin and encourages healthy testosterone levels. Vitamin B6 is critical for the biosynthesis of serotonin to help with relaxation. A terrific combination.

It is great that one of the easiest strategies to improve our health is by simply sleeping. When you sleep well, you will restore your balance to your life; you become more productive in your work and your workouts, and you can be of greater service to the world and those around you. Adequate amounts of sleep are critical to your overall health and lifestyle goals and the best part about it; it's free!

PART 2

HEALTHY = gutHEALTH

CHAPTER 7
Anti-Health: You Are What You Eat

"Food is fuel, not entertainment."

– Liz Nierzwicki

Like most people, I grew up on the standard American diet. The acronym for that diet is SAD, which is funny because it is a sad way of eating. I loved the quick and easy sugary filled packaged foods too. This SAD diet is loaded with man-made, boxed, processed foods with added sugar and chemicals that are made in laboratories.

Is something in a package actually food? I hardly think so. Food such as – plants, nuts, meats and fish, vegetables, and fruits – comes from the earth. I can't blame my mother for the diet I had as a child because she grew up in the uprising of the agricultural revolution and was heavily sold (like millions of other Americans) the idea of a low-fat high carbohydrate diet.

After studying nutrition science both in college and after, my education deepened and I learned the importance of whole foods and also how to cook great meals instead of buying the convenient but nutrient-poor packaged foods. The hardest part of my conversion from SAD to Paleo was that I had to undo years of taste bud programming and retrain my palate to like real foods; and on top of that, break the old habit of turning to convenient but nutrient-poor foods when in a time crunch.

How Our Eating Habits Deteriorated

"What is the agricultural revolution?" you ask. It is the transition from the Paleolithic diet, which consisted of real foods, to a diet consisting of cultivated man-made foods. The agricultural revolution was a period of great development and innovation. There was a massive increase in productivity and technology between the 18th century and the 19th century. It was, however, probably the worst thing that could have happened for human nutrition and brain evolution. With the changes in nutrition and gut health due to mass production of grains, our previously thriving and evolving ancestors began to decline. Research shows that early farmers who were eating grains were shorter than their hunter-gatherer ancestors - they did not live as long, they had smaller brains, and they also got many more infectious diseases and cavities.

Nearly all human illness and brain diseases are related to modern diet and can be prevented with proper nutrition. The human body evolved by eating natural and real foods that were hunted and gathered. Our ancestors ate seasonal plants and fruits, seeds, and hunted animals and fish and ate the entire animal.

The agricultural revolution introduced grains to the human digestive system – a system that didn't evolve with the enzymes to break down gluten or other parts of the plant. What I hear often from my clients and people who are generally healthy and not showing outward signs of distress after consuming grains – is that they don't feel they have a problem with them.

Grains have an array of chemical defenses as a natural part of the plant structure including various lectins, gluten, and phytic acid. These natural parts of the plant disrupt your human digestion, cause inflammation, and prevent you from absorbing vital nutrients and minerals. All grains contain some or all of these anti-nutrients. Because of what they do they are called anti-nutrients. An anti-nutrient is something that blocks and prevents nutrients from being absorbed by your body.

No wonder the early farmers who were eating mass produced grains had smaller brains and were shorter. They did not know it, but they were ingesting poisons. As our hunter-gatherer ancestors began eating grains more regularly, they no longer absorbed the nutrients and minerals needed to grow, develop, and maintain strong, healthy bodies.

A very large percentage of people are intolerant to gluten intolerant. Gluten is a substance that holds flour together in bread products and is present in a variety of grains. Gluten interferes with the body's ability to break down nutrients. When the body cannot break down food in the small intestine, inflammation happens and increases the risk of health and brain related issues such as mood disorders, migraines, seizures, muscle spasms, autism, Alzheimer's, celiac's disease, and the list goes on. Researchers in 2005 confirmed the effects of gluten on the brain due to their newfound knowledge of its inflammatory properties. Gluten sensitivities is not confined to the gut it always has an effect on the brain. Consumption of gluten causes a hormone response in the body that mimics the effects of opiates.

Many years after the boom of the agricultural revolution, came the low-fat diet craze. Up until the 1970s, the obesity rate in America had stayed fairly constant at around 12 percent of the adult population. In the 80s, things changed drastically. Obesity rates began a steady climb to where about 36 percent of the adult population is obese, and 74 percent are overweight, obese, or both. These numbers are still climbing to this day. With the help of new research, we are starting to realize that what we were told

- "fat and cholesterol are killing you" – is not true. It is the grains and sugars that we began to ingest that are detrimental to our health.

Through scientific research, we now know that when eaten in moderation, saturated fat has many positive side effects. We have learned that saturated fat encourages the liver cells to dump their fat cells, which helps the liver to function more effectively. Saturated fatty acids, especially the kinds found in butter and coconut, help white blood cells to recognize and destroy invading viruses and bacteria. Eating saturated fat tends to increase testosterone levels, which helps to repair tissue, preserve muscle, and improve sexual function for women and men alike.

When people started cutting out saturated fats from their diet, their health declined as well. When they cut out fats, they introduced more grains, more refined carbohydrates, and more sugar. My family jumped on this trend. We ate pasta, chips, candy corn (at Halloween), and low fat this and that, and we thought we were doing a great thing because we were not eating the fat. In reality, we were ruining our health. We were on a trajectory for ulcers, food allergies, irritable bowel syndrome, constipation, heart disease, and the list goes on.

The Consequences of Modern Diets

As a yoga studio owner, I come across people who are vegetarian, people who are vegan, and people who are still eating the standard American diet (processed foods). Many haven't even heard of the Paleo Diet. Those who are vegetarian or vegan choose these types of diets for a number of reasons. Usually, it's because they do not want to harm animals. I completely agree with this reason for going vegetarian. However, I come across many unhealthy vegetarian and vegans. Many run into health problems because they eat too much fruit, which can cause major insulin issues. Others simply miss out on many vitamins and minerals due to their limited diet.

Being vegetarian or vegan does not guarantee that you will be healthy or even healthier than individuals who consume saturated fats from animals. What matters is how you plan your vegetarian or vegan lifestyle. A vegetarian who consumes legumes, fruits, vegetables, seeds, and nuts will have a far different health profile than a vegetarian who has a diet that is high in refined carbohydrates like cookies, pasta, couscous, and muffins. In addition to that, a vegan or vegetarian diet can be lacking in certain key nutrients.

Any time you cut out a food group, there is a higher risk you could be missing out on certain nutrients such iron, calcium, vitamin B12, and zinc. Vitamin D and omega-3 fatty acid supplementation may also be necessary. In all actuality, these nutrients may be lacking in most people, and we all usually need supplementation. However, vegans and vegetarians may be missing considerable amounts of these vital nutrients.

The worst thing about the high-sugar eating regimen of a vegan, vegetarian, or someone eating the standard American diet is that it raises the body's insulin levels. When we eat too many carbohydrates, the pancreas pumps out insulin. When the liver and muscle cells are already filled with glycogen, which they normally are, those cells will eventually become resistant to the push of insulin. When glucose can't get into the muscle or liver cells, it remains in the bloodstream. This creates a problem because when the pancreas senses that there is still too much glucose in the blood, it will continue to pump out insulin. This excess insulin causes the insulin receptor sites on the surface of those cells to become more resistant because excess insulin is toxic in the blood-stream and it is trying to get rid of it. Eventually, the insulin helps the glucose to find its way into your fat cells, where it is stored as fat. It is not fat that is stored in your fat cells; it is sugar.

When a person consumes sugar or carbohydrates the blood sugar rises, insulin is released and there is a domino affect on the body: neurotransmitters that regulate mood are depleted, magnesium levels are diminished, vitamin B levels are depleted and glycation is increased.

As you continue to eat a high-carbohydrate diet and exercise less, the degree of insulin sensitivity increases. You will gain more and more weight, and your ability to lose weight will become extremely difficult.

To offset this, you need a dramatic shift in your diet by lowering our carbohydrate intake, increase healthy fats, dietary fiber, and proteins, and begin (or stick to) a strength-training program. Otherwise, you will develop several problems that will only get worse over time, and no amount of medicine will be able to fix it.

People need to understand that sugars (in all forms) are the most fattening and dangerous substance for the body. When you consume a lot of sugary foods, drinks, crackers, rice, or even fruits, you will have higher levels of glucose and therefore insulin in the blood and over time this will wreak havoc on the body.

Why Can't I Lose Weight?

If you've been a carbohydrate consumer and you cannot lose weight you may be experiencing insulin resistance. When you eat something sweet or when the body consumes carbohydrates you release insulin. This release of insulin causes the body's cells (particularly the muscle and fat cells) to absorb and use glucose from the blood. Insulin then binds to insulin receptor sites on the surface of the cells. When a person becomes insulin resistant because of the chronic drip of insulin from always consuming carbohydrates, the cells get to a point where they no longer allow the insulin to bind to the cell (they are resistant).

Insulin blocks the fat-burning enzyme lipase, so you can no longer burn fat. You continue to gain weight until the fat cells become resistant themselves. Next, the pancreas pumps out even more insulin because the body believes that what it already pumped out did not work, so it pumps more and more, making the situation even worse.

A communication breakdown has happened. Since the receptor sites are desensitized, they are no longer letting glucose into the muscle cells. This breakdown also prevents amino acids (protein) from entering, which then causes your body to turn to your hard-earned muscle to break down essential amino acids into glucose and use that as energy. This is a severe break-down of cells and not the way the body is meant to operate. In addition, you can't build or maintain your muscles.

When we are in this catabolic state, we experience low levels of energy. We feel as if we are hungry all the time, and we crave carbohydrates. We then have no desire to work out because we are tired, and the cycle continues.

On top of that, when your liver becomes insulin resistant, it can no longer convert thyroid hormone T4 into the T3. As a result, you then begin to have "thyroid problems," which further slow your metabolism. Eventually, the pancreas burns out. Then you can't produce any more insulin, and you get insulin-dependent Type 2 diabetes.

What Can We Do About It?

Healthy eating habits and an understanding the gut (small intestines) microbiome is essential to avoiding all of the above. We will discuss how the gut works in further detail in the next chapter. You can gain more knowledge and establish healthy habits by using the figureFIT! Paleo Food Guide located in the back of the book. It will show you what we eat on the figureFIT! Program. As you cut back on bad carbohydrates and start training your energy systems via the figureFIT! workouts, you will notice that your health problems begin to go away, your energy levels rise, and your sleep improves.

The good news is that solving the problem, at least on an individual level, is easy. So why not start there? We can repair the systems in our bodies by eating real foods again. Draw a line in the sand. Give up sugar. Throw out the packaged foods and resolve to not buy them again – not for you, your kids, or any cookout or party that you attend. Promise yourself that you will begin to eat real foods again. You will cut out the processed cookies and boxed foods and begin to eat the egg yolks (loaded with vitamins), bacon again (who doesn't want bacon?), and tons of vegetables.

Your money speaks volumes, and you will create a demand for what you are willing to support. Use your dollars wisely and support only organic and ethical farming practices. Too much animal cruelty is happening in our country today, and change must happen. When you purchase non-organic and mass-produced foods, you are choosing to support those farming practices. Choose your foods wisely.

CHAPTER 8
Digestive Disorders and Problems

"Let food be thy medicine and medicine be thy food."

– Hippocrates

Up to 80 percent of the immune system is in the gut! If you eat things that are bad for you, then no wonder you are tired and sick, have rashes and allergies, are overweight, or have other chronic problems. Even if you eat clean food, there still might be a problem with something that you eat, so it is worth looking into.

Most problems start with inflammation. Inflammation can either be acute (short term) or chronic (long term). Acute inflammation is your body's short-term response to damage. The body begins to heal itself quickly. Chronic inflammation is ongoing or long-term inflammation that causes more breakdown of tissue than the body can rebuild. Chronic inflammation stretches the inflammatory response out over months or years, which creates all sorts of problems.

Signs of Digestive Disorders:

- Constipation or diarrhea
- Gas after meals
- Chronic conditions such as asthma, rheumatoid arthritis, or osteoporosis

- Any other problem after eating
- Chronic Candida infections, which can cause skin rashes and vaginal yeast infections in women.
- Undigested food in stool
- Known or unknown food sensitivities
- Indigestion or belching after meals
- Frequent upset stomach
- Frequent sickness
- Frequent fatigue
- Skin rashes
- Extra weight on the body

Some other problems from digestion are shown in the following table:

Acid reflux	Acne	Allergies	Anemia
Arthritis	Asthma	Bronchitis	Bursitis
Cancer	Celiac Disease	Chronic Pain	Circulation Issues
Colitis	Crohn's Disease	Dementia	Depression
Dermatitis	Diabetes 1 & 2	Eczema	Edema
Endometriosis	Fibromyalgia	Gout	Grave's Disease
Hashimoto	Heart Disease	High Blood Pressure	High Cholesterol
Infertility	IBS	Insulin Resistance	Joint Pain
Lupus	Migraines	Multiple Sclerosis	Obesity
Raynaud's	Seizures	Tendonitis	Vasculitis

The Gut

The gut consists of the small intestine and the colon (large intestine). There is immune tissue that follows the entire length of your small intestine. The small intestine is where most of your food is broken down into usable form such as amino acids (from protein), fatty acids (from fat), glucose (from carbohydrates), vitamins, and minerals. If you suffer from a digestive disorder or a malfunction in the gut, the food might *not* be used properly. Instead, it might be recognized as an enemy to the system, and this is called "leaky gut syndrome."

On top of its [the intestines] many folds are forests of tiny fingershaped protrusions called villae. Together, the folds and the villae make the gut's surface area as big as two tennis courts.[14]

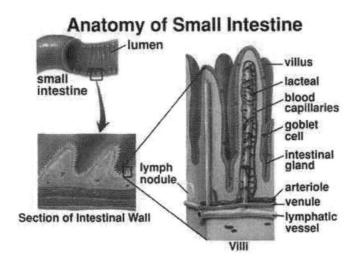

15

The digestive system works by propelling food through the intestines over 24 hours. Muscle contractions squeeze the food through the different sections of the intestine that are separated by bands of muscles, or sphincters, that act as valves.

---

[14] Anatomy of the gut - Medtronic. (n.d.). Retrieved August 12, 2015, from http://www.medtronic-gastro-uro.com.au/bowel-anatomy-of-the-gut.html

[15] Small Intestine. (n.d.). Retrieved August 12, 2015, from http://missinglink.ucsf.edu/lm/IDS_106_LowerGI/Lower%20GI/mainpages/ smallintestine.htm

The passage of food from one area of the intestines to another is coordinated so that food stays in a specific area for long enough for the gut to absorb fluids and nutrients, or process and expel waste.[16]

Leaky Gut Syndrome. Leaky gut syndrome is now being understood as a real condition that affects millions of people. The lining of your digestive tract is like a net with extremely small holes (when not leaky) in it that only allow specific substances to pass through. Your gut lining works as a barrier keeping out bigger particles that can damage your system. The theory is that leaky gut syndrome (also called increased intestinal permeability), is the result of damage to the intestinal lining, making it inflamed allowing, undigested particles, bacteria, and other toxins into the blood stream. This triggers an autoimmune reaction, which can lead to gastrointestinal problems such as abdominal bloating, excessive gas and cramps, fatigue, food sensitivities, joint pain, skin rashes, and autoimmune problems.

Leaky gut syndrome may trigger or worsen such disorders as Crohn's disease, celiac disease, rheumatoid arthritis, and asthma.[17]

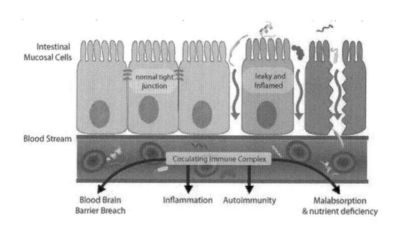

[16] Anatomy of the gut - Medtronic. (n.d.). Retrieved August 12, 2015, from http://www.medtronic-gastro-uro.com.au/bowel-anatomy-of-the-gut.html
[17] Q & A Library. (n.d.). Retrieved August 12, 2015, from http:// www.drweil.com/drw/u/QAA361058/what-is-leaky-gut.html

Another Major Problem: Small Intestinal Bacterial Overgrowth

Small intestinal bacteria overgrowth, also known in the health community as SIBO, is a condition in which bacteria in the small intestine has overgrown and become problematic. Lack of movement in the small intestine, areas of obstruction, or non-draining pockets (called diverticuli) can be a source of this overgrowth.

SIBO symptoms include (but are not limited to):

- Abdominal bloating
- Abdominal pain
- Abdominal cramps
- Gas
- Diarrhea
- Constipation
- Heartburn/GERD
- Nausea
- Candida

Some likely and common causes of SIBO include:

- Food poisoning (especially during foreign travel)
- Exposure to contaminated water
- Pathogens
- Previous surgery involving the small intestine
- Medications, including antibiotics and pain relievers (NSAIDS)
- Conditions that reduce gut motility
- Other health conditions, such as celiac disease

SIBO compromises the basic structure and function of the small intestine. The bacteria feed on what you eat, robbing you of nutrients as well as fermenting the food, drawing water into the small intestine, and causing bloating, gas, pain, and the other symptoms listed previously.[18]

Bacterial overgrowth in the small intestine can lead to damage of the lining of the small intestine therefore causing leaky gut and leaky gut can then lead to a host of other issues such as:

- Fibromyalgia
- Parkinson's disease
- Chronic renal failure
- Hypothyroidism
- Rheumatoid arthritis
- Liver disease
- Scleroderma
- Pancreatic insufficiency
- Diverticulosis
- Diabetes
- Crohn's disease
- Celiac disease
- Rosacea
- Restless leg syndrome

Consider the Following Questions:

- Does your energy fluctuate throughout the day?

---

[18] Sanfilippo, D. (n.d.). Retrieved August 12, 2015, from http:// balancedbites.com/wp-content/uploads/2014/05/ SimplifyingSIBO_ BalancedBites.pdf

- How do you feel most of the time?

- How much fat do you have compared to muscle?

- How is your appetite?

- Do you crave certain things such as sugar, salt, or fatty foods?

- Does your skin have rashes often or chronically on the back of your arm?

- Is your skin healthy, clear, and glowing?

- Do you suffer problems are eating certain foods?

- Do you have regular bowel movements?

- Do you have IBS?

- How is your dental health and vision?

- How is your energy?

- Do you have yeast or Candida?

- How are your moods?

The Price to Pay for Unhealthy Habits

In college, I would party and drink with my friends. And like any college kids, when we came back late at night, we would order in. We got pizza, soda, and breadsticks with that awful nacho cheese that is loaded with partially hydrogenated oils and virtually no real cheese. I never liked the idea of eating that food late at night, so I got the bright idea (not a good idea at all) to take a laxative so that I would get rid of everything that I had eaten the next morning. It was my form of bulimia. Little did I know that I was slowly ruining my bowel.

While I was in college, I took nutrition classes, and I started to learn about how the body burns calories. I learned that we burn carbohydrates first, then fats, and then protein. I also learned that when we eat a lot of carbohydrates, we don't burn any fat. So if we try to lose weight, and all we eat is carbohydrates, we won't lose any fat.

Around the same time, Dr. Atkins' diet became popular. People cut out carbohydrates and ate all the protein they wanted. The problem was that people were not eating enough vegetables. They were eating protein and losing weight, but they got into cycles where they craved other foods since their diet lacked balance. As a result, many people who did the Atkins diet rebounded back to their heavy weight. The diet got a bad rap because people weren't doing it right. They were eating meat, cheese, and high-saturated fatty foods only. Those who ate vegetables and relatively low saturated fatty foods did extremely well with this diet.

As part of my education, I went to study international marketing in Finland before my senior year. It was quite an eye-opener in many ways. One way was how Americans eat. The grocery stores in Finland were about a quarter of the size of the grocery stores in the United States. They did not have the 20 aisles of boxed food that we have. They had produce, meat, and one or two aisles with packaged items, mainly house-hold necessities, and that was it. They didn't have the aisles and aisles of processed foods that I was familiar with. Mac & cheese was a staple for me, and I didn't find that there.

I realized that I would not be able to eat what I was used to eating. At the time, I did not care as much about food as I do now, so I bought some of the things that I knew I could eat like chicken, vegetables, and apples. I figured I would learn to like the local food. However, once I tried it, I was unimpressed. The salads were shredded cabbage, and for a girl who was used to iceberg and spinach, this was weird food to me, so I shunned it.

Luckily for me, there was a McDonald's in town. I wasn't interested in eating McDonald's food in the least bit, and I knew that it was awful for me. But I would eat it on occasion because I knew what to expect. I also had a ton of ice cream. They had a little ice cream stand in the center of the market. I would often purchase the ice cream and call it a day. I called my mom and asked her to send me a care package. She shipped me Mac & cheese, tuna, and Cheetos – the complete standard American cuisine. In other words, my diet was extremely unhealthy while I was there. In addition to the bad food, I would have nightly drinks with the crew.

Remember my laxative days back in the states? Well, that ruined me. I got to a point where I could no longer go to the bathroom. I didn't know it at the time, but taking laxatives that way stopped my bowel from doing its job. I was now dependent on the laxatives, but I did not have them there and had no idea where I could buy any.

I would run in the morning because I knew that could help my body move things along, but it didn't help at all. In desperation, I emailed my mom, and she sent prune juice from the United States. But all it did was give me awful gas and bloat my stomach. Nothing worked. I could not go to the bathroom and began to experience pain right above my right hipbone. I felt pressure, and all I could imagine was how full of shit I was – literally. I'm laughing now because I'm healed, but at the time it was not fun or funny.

In thirteen weeks, I had only one bowel movement. I was in a lot of pain, and when I came back to the States, I knew I had to go to the doctor immediately.

When I got to the doctor, the doctor said that I either had a blockage, or there was something else going on in my digestive system. He said that I would have to take something from the bottom up and the top down to clear myself out. If that didn't work, there could be something more serious going on. My doctor was cool about it and made a joke that I would be about 5 pounds lighter after the whole excavation process. He thought that was quite funny, but I didn't because I was the one dealing with the pain, and I just wanted my body to work again.

After the process of clearing out my body, the doctor found out that I did not have a blockage, and there was nothing else wrong with me. I just needed to get my colon working again. It had stopped working because of all the laxatives I had been taking; it had become dependent on the laxatives.

My prescription was to drink a lot of water, exercise daily, and eat a lot of fiber, mainly spinach and vegetables. I slowly started going to the bathroom again, but it was not perfect. It was maybe every two days, and for a long time, that was my new normal. But every two days is not good enough either, and I know this now. Ideally, we should be going after every time we eat or multiple times in one day, *not* every other day.

Flash forward sixteen years, now that same Doctor is referring patients to me to help get their bowels working again. Constipation is a big issue in the United States, and I would say that it's a big issue even on a global scale. Patients who need help in this area are referred to in order to help them get on a nutrition plan that makes their body function optimally again, or for some, for the first time in their life.

After my studies in nutrition, I continued my journey to learn as much as I could about nutrition and health. After I graduated college and started working in the corporate world, nutrition and fitness became my first hobby. Acting and modeling was my second.

Once I started to dig deeper into the world of information about nutrition, I began to realize that many of the problems I was experiencing, such as breathing issues, allergies, and even yeast infections, could be due to the foods I was eating.

I started to pay attention to how I would feel after eating certain foods. Sometimes it would become difficult for me to breathe after drinking diet soda or eating certain packaged candies or crackers. Sugary foods seemed to deplete my energy and make me tired. I noticed that when I would binge on cookies or something sweet, I would later get crabby or irritable.

At the same time, I was becoming a yoga teacher. My yoga teacher told me about how they had tested her blood to find out what food her body was building antibodies to. I wanted to take the same test, so I got my blood taken, and they looked at the full spectrum of foods, additives, and dyes. I learned that my body was building antibodies to many foods, and some of the additives in food, such as dyes, were highly problematic to my body. They told me to cut the foods and dyes out of my diet for six weeks, and then I could reintroduce them one at a time to see how my body reacted.

Some foods I did not even want to reintroduce because they were not good for me. Around that same time, in 2011, I learned about the Paleo diet, the Paleolithic diet. It is the food that our ancestors evolved on. They ate nuts, seeds, and vegetables. They hunted for food, and they ate most parts of the animals they caught.

The Paleo diet mentioned cutting out bread and dairy because of the host of problems that they can cause. It was a process for me because I was always snacking on crackers, and I loved to make sandwiches. As I cut these out, my body started feeling better. My every three-day bowel movement started to increase to daily bowel movements. My terrible eye allergies that I used to have disappeared. Once I cut grains and dairy out of my diet, those problems went away and haven't returned. My sleeping and breathing have improved, and I started to slim down, all because I got rid of the food that was problematic for my body.

When I tell my clients that it took me about two years to fully get rid of gluten and wheat from my diet, it makes them feel better about their lapses. What took me longer was my sweet tooth. Some people have salty cravings; I tend to have sugary cravings. I found that when I am eating a balanced diet, I have fewer cravings. I also found that during my monthly cycle, I crave sugary foods for one week. If I'm not aware of where I'm at in my cycle and plan accordingly to drink extra water and eat clean foods, I will go through the kitchen like Mrs. Pac-man.

When you transition from a SAD diet to a Paleo Diet, I suggest replacing foods instead of eliminating something completely. Don't just go cold turkey. If you love milk, substitute it with almond milk or coconut milk. If you like bread, substitute it with homemade Paleo bread. If you're a soda drinker, substitute the soda with carbonated lemon water. For a while, after going Paleo, I continued to eat cereal because I loved it, and it was easy. I thought I could make one exception by eating a "gluten free" cereal. However, when you go on the Paleo diet, it's important to give your body the chance to show you how healthy it *can* be by fully eliminating the foods that are known to cause problems. The kicker for me was when I found out that the only cereal I would eat – the Kashi brand – got slammed in the media because they had genetically modified ingredients. Then I decided I was done; I quit eating cereal. A few short weeks later, my body became even more regular, and my energy became fantastic. There was something to this Paleo thing.

What It Really Is About: gutHEALTH

After two years of being on the Paleo diet, I was finally regular with my bowel movements. But I got into the habit of eating too many Paleo treats and things that turned into sugar in my digestive system. My staples were broccoli, asparagus, apples, and meats. However, due to the imbalance of eating the same foods over and over again, and because of this, creating an out-of-balance gut microbiome, I started getting monthly yeast infections.

The human gut microbiome is located mainly in our small intestines. This is where the food is broken down and absorbed (or not) for the body's use.

The human microbiome is composed of bacteria, archaea, viruses, and eukaryotic microbes that reside in and on our bodies. These microbes have tremendous potential to impact our physiology, both in health and in disease. They contribute to metabolic functions, protect against pathogens, educate the immune system, and, through these basic functions, affect directly or indirectly most of our physiological functions.[19]

The study of the human microbiome has been furthered by technological advancements. Studies on the function of the microbiota will be critical to understanding the role of the microbiota in human homeostasis [and how diseases are formed or destroyed].[20]

---

[19] Shreiner, A., Kao, J., & Young, V. (2015, January 31). Med-scape Log In. Retrieved August 13, 2015, from http://www.medscape.com/viewarticle/837078

[20] Grice, E., & Segre, J. (2012, June 6). The Human Microbiome: Our Second Genome. Retrieved August 13, 2015, from http://www. ncbi.

My OBGYN doctor told me that the infections were most likely come from my clothes being sweaty after my workout or after teaching hot yoga. She advised me to change quicker into dry clothes.

However, I did not believe that it was my sweat that caused the infections. With my knowledge of food and awareness that the smallest thing can cause a problem, I just knew that it came from something I was eating. I dove in and did more research. I learned about the gut microbiome and started to research foods again.

Then I learned about FODMAPs. FODMAP stands for fermentable oligosaccharides, disaccharides, monosaccharides, and polyols. FODMAPs are foods that are poorly absorbed in the small intestine, which means they can be left there to ferment. For that reason, they can cause the symptoms of IBS, candida, and other health issues. I found out about a low FODMAP diet that was developed to treat irritable bowel syndrome and control other gastrointestinal disorders, so I put myself on a low FODMAP diet. After I started this diet, I didn't have any more symptoms of candida. I was finally beginning to understand my gut health and realized that it goes way beyond just eating the Paleo way; we actually have to eat for the health of our gut. This understanding put me on a path to healing. *Finally*.

You do not need to go through all of the expensive tests to determine what food you can eat like I did. It's actually easy to eat healthy and clean. What I suggest in the beginning is simply transitioning over to eating real whole foods. If you still eat grains, cut them out of your diet. There is no reason to eat them. Remember that they contain anti-nutrients. If you eat dairy, switch to coconut milk or almond milk.

Once you eat real foods again and eat a balanced diet, you should find that your health greatly improves. Most illnesses and diseases can be cured with proper nutrition; so don't underestimate the power of good quality earth given foods. Sometimes eating healthy (for you) may go beyond just eating real foods like it was for me. Sometimes you need to

nlm.nih.gov/pmc/articles/PMC3518434/

cut out a certain category of foods like I had to with FODMAPS. Once you have eaten the foods listed on the figureFIT! Paleo Food Guide for six to eight weeks, see where you're at with your health. If you still need more support to manage your gut health, you can reach out to my team and me.

Every cell in the body is constantly dying, and new cells are being remade with the foods we consume, the air we breathe, and the hormones that we are releasing. After approximately three weeks, the cells of the gut die off, and new cells are made. This is why it is suggested to eat the Paleo way for approximately six weeks before you decide it is working or not for you. Once you cut out the harmful foods from your diet, your body will rapidly start to heal. Just give it time and put your whole heart into the process.

CHAPTER 9
The figure*FIT!* Nutrition Plan

"When you are triggered, that is simply a red flag to a place that needs understanding, self-love, and often times forgiveness."

– Liz Nierzwicki

Think differently than the rest. Learn your emotional triggers around food. Let your nutrition be a way you fuel your body for optimal health, not a way to fuel your feelings. Have such a deep conviction about your nutrition that when you walk past the cinnamon rolls in the mall, you enjoy the smell, but you don't even think twice about buying one. It may take you time to get to this mindset, but when you are eating for optimal gut health and mental health and a peak fitness level, you will no longer crave such awful foods. You will be aware that it is an empty calorie that does nothing for you other than harm you.

The pleasure we gain from eating something that tastes good (yet is bad for us) does not last long. What does last long are the effects of what we eat: stored fat, energy crashes, guilt, negative self-talk, diabetes, overgrowth of bad bacteria in the gut, and the list goes on.

Food is fuel. It's important to begin to think beyond the cravings and old habits. Your nutrition needs to become a way of life for you. Eat proper foods for the right reasons and at the right times. Eat for optimal health functioning and not to fuel your emotions.

The figureFIT! Lifestyle Program is all about eating for optimal health and energy levels. The foods we eat are real foods – vegetables, meat, fruit, nuts, and healthy oils. We choose to feed our bodies foods that are rich in nutrients and loaded with natural vitamins and minerals. We stay away from foods that are "empty" and do not provide us with nutrition. We are careful about where our foods come from, and we try to buy local organic produce and meat as often as possible.

This is not by any means a diet; it's a lifestyle that will help you stay healthy, fit, and feeling great. When we aim for well-balanced nutrition and feed our body high-quality (organic) meats, vegetables, fruits, and healthy fats like avocado, coconut, and olive oil, we stay satisfied. Our cravings for unhealthy sugary foods will reduce, and we will crave the foods that are good for us.

I remember the first time I did a sugar detox. After five days, I had an awful headache. This is called the healing crisis. As the body is getting back to an appropriate homeostasis, it may sometimes go through detox-like symptoms. After day six, I started feeling great. My energy spiked, I craved salads, and I was more alert than ever. I knew instantly that the sugar detox was one of the best things I could have done for myself.

Eating real food allows us to maintain balanced energy and a healthy metabolism, and it keeps our immune system healthy. The figureFIT! eating style is good for your energy levels, sleep quality, mood, attention span, and quality of life. This type of eating style will help you eliminate binge eating, sugar cravings, and other unhealthy food patterns. Perhaps the biggest benefit of all is that it can *minimize* our risk for food-related diseases such as diabetes, cardiovascular diseases, stroke, and autoimmune conditions.

Bonus: Once you start feeling better and see your body changing, your old food desires will fall away. As you begin to feel good in your new clothes and love the way you look and feel, you won't want to eat foods that take you away from these good feelings. You'll become addicted to the way this type of lifestyle makes you feel.

Food Facts

Food is made up of micronutrients (vitamins, minerals, antioxidants, and phytochemicals) and macronutrients (energy). Macronutrients are proteins, fats, and carbohydrates.

Carbohydrates

- They are the body's cheap fuel source.

- They provide energy for activity and fuel for the brain.

- There are four calories in 1 gram of carbohydrate.

- A salivary enzyme called amylase breaks down carbohydrates into sugar. Starches are converted into glucose and absorbed in the small intestine. Then they are pushed into the bloodstream where they become blood glucose.

- Excess is stored as fat.

Proteins

- Protein provides the building blocks of every cell in the body, muscles, connective tissues, bones, skin, and hair.

- Protein is needed for growth, repair, and recovery.

- Protein amino acids are used to produce hormones, enzymes, neurotransmitters, DNA/RNA, and antibodies.

- There are four calories per 1 gram of protein.

- Protein breaks down into amino acids while they are in the small intestine. They are held there until amino acids can be absorbed across the gut lining into the bloodstream.

Fats

- Fats are a dense source of energy.

- They are necessary to absorb the fat-soluble vitamins A, D, E, and K.

- They provide satiety when they are eaten with protein.

- Healthy fats are needed to insulate nerve fibers and help transmit nerve impulses.

- Fat helps to transport nutrients and metabolites across cell membranes.

- They help to develop healthy sex hormones and immune functioning.

- There are nine calories per 1 gram of fat.

- Fat is broken down into fatty acids and glycerol upon digestion. The majority of digestion occurs in the small intestine and stays there until the fat crosses the intestinal lining into the blood-stream.

- Fat slows down the digestion/absorption process of carbohydrates and proteins and helps to keep you full longer.

What to Eat

The foods we eat on the figureFIT! Lifestyle Program are foods that were available to the first inhabitants of the earth through hunting and gathering such as meat and fish, nuts and seeds, fruits, and vegetables. In this lifestyle, we avoid processed, refined, and nutrition-deficient foods such as grains, dairy, and other man-made foods. These foods are difficult for the body to digest and cause many problems seen and unseen.

The figureFIT! Paleo Food Guide at the back of the book will provide you with a list of foods recommended and considered to be optimal for digestion, blood sugar regulation, metabolism, and long-lasting energy. On the figureFIT! Lifestyle Program, you will eat foods from:

- Properly farmed organic meat – enjoy meat from grass-fed, pasture-raised, organically fed animals.

- Free range poultry and eggs – best if it is local and free-range.

- Fish from sustainable fishing practices – wild-caught fish are best because it means that they were caught in the wild and not farm-raised.

- Vegetables and fruits – no one ever got fat eating vegetables. Some vegetables are best enjoyed organic, and others are not necessary to buy organic. Fruits should be eaten as a dessert and not with a meal because they can be bad for your blood sugar. If you are looking to lose weight, I encourage you to limit your fruit intake and keep blood sugar levels stable.

- Healthy fats and oils – choose the best quality fats you can find that will help you on your fitness journey. Go to The figureFIT! Paleo Food Guide in the back of the book for more information on healthy fats and oils.

- Nuts and seeds – this is an easy snack but can easily be overdone as nuts and seed are dense in calories. If your goal is fat loss, make sure you abide by portion sizes. In addition, some nuts are better for you than others. The figureFIT! Paleo Food Guide will offer you suggestions on which nuts are best.

What Not to Eat

When I was allergy tested for foods via a blood draw to see what my body was building antibodies too, I found I was highly allergic to food additives more than any food. I searched and searched for where a specific additive was coming from, and I couldn't find it. As a result, I decided to cut out all boxed foods and anything else that had ingredients in which I didn't know what they were. Bottom line, if it is in a package or man-made with more than three ingredients, the chances are that you should not be eating it. I'm often asked what should I avoid. Here is my quick list:

- Refined and whole grains – yes, you read that right! This includes baked goods, cereal, bread, English muffins, pasta, pita bread, bagels, wheat, barley, rye, spelt, corn, buckwheat, millet, etc.

- Processed food and meal replacement bars – crackers, cookies, pretzels, chips, breakfast bars, granola bars, toaster pastries, snack bars, etc.

- Pasteurized dairy – processed and pasteurized milk, cheese, yogurt, cottage cheese, ice cream, frozen yogurt, etc. Raw dairy might be allowed *if* you can find good raw, grass-fed milk and cheese from a local farmer and your body is okay after eating it.

- Soy – soy contains plant estrogens in the form of isoflavones, which disrupt your body's hormones and will throw everything out of balance. Soy and grains also contain *lectins*. If you mess with your leptin sensitivity, aka your hunger and energy expenditure signals, it can make you think you are hungry when you are not, therefore, causing weight gain. Leptin resistance also leads to insulin resistance, which can cause metabolic syndrome, leading to diabetes, heart disease, stroke, weight gain, etc. In addition to lectins, soy and grains also have *phytates.* Phytates bind to minerals that your body needs, such as zinc, magnesium, calcium, and iron, making them unavailable to for your body to absorb them. "There's also substantial evidence that soy, in its processed form (i.e. soy milk, soy protein isolate, etc.) is an endocrine disruptor and anti-nutrient and is best avoided."[21]

---

[21] Beyond Paleo: Food fascism and the 80/20 rule. (2013, December 17). Retrieved August 12, 2015, from http://chriskresser.com/beyond-paleo-12/

- Refined sugar – refined sugar is a poison to the body because it has been depleted of all its vitamins and minerals. It is an empty calorie that lacks the natural minerals that are present in the sugar beet or cane. Sugar drains the body of precious vitamins and minerals because of its damage to the digestive system. Also, when you eat sugary foods, you start a sugar craving cycle that is hard to break. Sugar robs energy and lowers your immune system.

- Sweetened beverages – Anything artificially sweetened will wreak havoc on your system. Completely avoid anything artificially sweetened such as soda, energy drinks, juice, teas, coffee drinks, smoothies, etc.

- Alcohol will halt your efforts because when you drink alcohol, your liver stops metabolizing fats, and everything you eat around drinking gets stored as fat. Alcohol will also impair your decision-making skills. Who goes home after a night of drinking and eats chicken and broccoli? See what I mean? When you do drink, make the decision that you will only have one or two drinks and stick with it. Make a hard and fast rule about how you will behave around drinking and what you will eat before and after. Before and after you drink, it's important that you eat plenty of veggies and avoid high amounts of fats around the time you drink.

How Do We Fix Our Digestive System?

I am a firm believer that, for the most part, the figureFIT! Nutrition Plan is the best nutrition for our bodies because it is based on wholesome real foods that are earth given and not man-made. However, when someone comes to me, and they deal with multiple health problems, we put them on a strict figureFIT! Low-FODMAP Diet for a short period. As Chris Kresser said,

It gives us a baseline to work from. By removing all common food toxins and observing what happens, we learn which foods may be contributing to their issues and to what extent. Then the next steps usually become a lot more clear.[22]

I feel that a few of nature's foods are missing from the figureFIT! Paleo Food Guide such as legumes (beans and peanuts) and potatoes. Some foods are more harmful than others such as *wheat, sugar, high-fructose corn syrup, and industrial seed oils.* These foods have been proven to be toxic to the body and contribute to virtually all modern diseases from heart disease, to diabetes and obesity. For the most part, the figureFIT! Program excludes potatoes and legumes (beans and peanuts) due to the distress that they put on the gut for some people. However, recent research by Stephan Guyenet revealed that it is quite possible to eat potatoes and be perfectly healthy. The same goes for legumes; many healthy vegetarians have been relying on them for a major part of their diet for decades.

Once you start eating the figureFIT! way, you will notice results quickly. You will find that after just a few days, your energy levels will start to stabilize and you will have fewer sugar cravings. Once you've been eating this way for a few weeks and months, your allergies will start to go away, your immune system will get stronger, your auto-immune responses will start to subside, and you may even need to buy new clothes due to loss of excess weight.

After going Paleo, my health changed significantly. I used to get sinus infections every year, and I used to take Advair and other bronchial dilators to help me breathe better. Also, my eyes used to get extremely itchy and red, and I would need special eye drops. In addition, I always used to be constipated and in need of some stool softener or bowel-producing supplement. It was horrible. I didn't know that something as

---

[22] Beyond Paleo: Food fascism and the 80/20 rule. (2013, December 17). Retrieved August 12, 2015, from http://chriskresser.com/beyond-paleo-12/

simple as cutting out certain foods (that I didn't even like) could help. When I cut out the SAD foods, my health changed drastically. Now I no longer have any of these problems. They are like a distant bad dream.

It's easy to eat the right way. Do yourself a favor: Stop telling yourself how much you love certain foods and how you can't live without them, and take my program that helps break bad habits.

I love when I find myself attached to certain things because I love beating my bad habits and *breaking* them. I deploy my bad habit breaking measures to break my bad habits or attachment to things that I have suddenly become addicted to. Find my figureFIT! Worksheet III: "Breaking Bad Habits" in the back of the book and use it anytime you find yourself attaching to something. Even if it is something that may be good for you, know that there needs to be balance in everything you do.

If you are currently following a standard American diet, then start by eliminating *all* the foods in the "avoid" section of the Daily Food Target Guide (located in the back of the book), and pay attention to how you feel. If you become a member of the program, start trying the many recipes on the site, and give it 30 days before you assess what is going on internally. Realistically, it takes about three to six weeks to start seeing changes.

figure*FIT!* Food Rules and Guidelines

1. Always eat your macronutrients. This is the amount of proteins, carbohydrates, and healthy fats that your body needs daily. The ratios might change based on your goals, but you need to hit your caloric intake daily. If you would like more help learning about your macro-nutrient profile, head to figurefitlife.com/shop and sign up to get your macronutrient profile.

2. *Always* have a breakfast with protein and good fats, not any sugar. This will give you proper energy and a level head for the rest of your day. Breakfasts loaded with sugar throw off your energy and mind for the whole day.

3. Base your meals around *protein*. The serving size of the protein should be the size of your palm. Try to choose protein from the "best" category from the Daily Food Target Guide or preferably from the figureFIT! Paleo Food Guide.

4. Fill the rest of your plate with *vegetables*.

5. *Fruit* is meant to be a treat or eaten after a workout to restore lost glycogen. Fruit should not take the place of vegetables at meals nor should it be your primary source of carbohydrates. Choose fruits that are low in sugar as often as possible, and choose from the "best and better" list in the Daily Food Target Guide or preferably from the figureFIT! Paleo Food Guide.

6. Eat healthy *fats and oils*. Do not skimp of fats because you think they will make you fat; that is one of the biggest errors you could make. Fats and oils are needed for the brain and the nervous system and the production of energy and most of the body's vital hormones. Your body *needs* healthy fats and oils to transport vitamins, minerals, and hormones in and out of every cell in the body. Omega-3's EPA and DHA are two essential fatty acids needed to have a healthy nervous system. They can be obtained from quality fish, sardines, and fish oils.

7. *Stay away from sugar.* Sugary foods, such as cakes, man-made desserts, pies, sugary drinks, cookies, etc., should be avoided 95 percent of the time. Sugar robs the body of vitamins and minerals, lowering your immune system and making you susceptible to frequent colds, digestive disorders, autoimmune disorders, diabetes, and a host of other issues. Save sugary treats for special occasions. If you are a sugar addict and need to cut the chord, sign up for "The Game Changer," which is a one-month sugar detox that will help you rid of the habit for good.

Meal Planning

Practice good mealtime habits. Eat meals at the table, not in front of the TV or while you are on the phone. When you are distracted, you will eat more. Take the time to eat your meal so that your body is responsive to the clues your body is sending.

Daily meals: Eat three to five meals per day. Start with a good breakfast. Base each meal around one palm-sized protein source. Fill the rest of your plate with vegetables. A serving of healthy fat should be added to each meal.

If you need snacks in between each meal, base your snack around a protein and balance it out with a fat (like 1 serving of almonds) or vegetables.

Fruit should be eaten around workouts, either before or after your workout.

Pre-workout: If you exercise early in the morning, you can do cardio on an empty stomach *only* if your body is okay with that. Some people need food before they exercise. But when you eat, your blood goes right to the stomach for digestion and will not be available to your muscles right away, so give yourself about one hour to digest. If you eat carbohydrates, your body will not need to turn to stored body fat to create glucose because you will have just fed that to your body. Therefore, eating carbohydrates before working out eliminates any fat burning. If you are going to exercise in the morning, it is best to either eat only protein 45-60 minutes prior *or* do cardio first and eat immediately after working out.

Post-workout: Eat immediately after your workouts (within 30 minutes). This meal should be protein and a fast digesting carbohydrate to replenish glycogen. Have *no* fat at this meal.

The post-workout meal is a bonus meal and not meant to replace breakfast, lunch, or dinner. It is a necessary source of fuel designed to help you recover faster from high-intensity exercise.

Eating the proper amount of macronutrients daily is critical to our overall health. If we eat too much, we will gain weight. If we eat too little (consistently), the body will think we are starving and will start to store body fat.

We've now discussed that the type of food you eat matters. We have seen that what we eat breaks down into micronutrients (vitamins and minerals), and if we eat the proper foods, we will be fueled correctly.

Often, due to time restraints or simply not wanting to eat another meal, I supplement with meal replacement shakes. I have been taking Isagenix meal replacements shakes for years. I searched high and low for high-quality meal replacement shakes, and I could not find any that tasted good until I found Isagenix. (IsaLean Shake: Natural Berry Harvest) from Isagenix. This meal replacement shake is the perfect balance of protein and carbohydrates to refuel my body after one of my workouts. I'm a big proponent of meal replacement shakes to help get in the body's proper amount of protein. If you're interested in meal replacement supplements to help you achieve your total daily caloric intake, check out my Isagenix site: liznierzwicki.isagenix.com

Check out the Meal Planning Guide at the back of the book on how to build your meals throughout your day.

CHAPTER 10
Becoming A Fat-Burning Machine

Would you love to burn the fat right off your body and then remain at your ideal body weight for the rest of your life? It is much easier than we have made it over the last hundreds of years.

The body is built to optimize stored body fat for fuel. When we load the body full of carbohydrates, we are not doing ourselves any justice. In fact, we are slowly killing ourselves. The human body evolved on a hunter-gatherer diet filled with plenty of plants and proteins – not the chronic glucose drip that you see in today's (anti) nutrition culture.

Over the years, food companies and uneducated people have been telling us that we need carbohydrates. The fact of the matter is we do not need that many carbohydrates. The body does not need or want more than one teaspoon of glucose in the bloodstream at any given time. I'll repeat that, the body does not need or want more than one teaspoon of glucose at any given time. If it does it will do what it can to get it out of the system and it does that by releasing insulin and storing the excess in the cells. THIS is what makes us fat. The body works optimally when it has adequate amounts of protein (amino acids for cell building) and fat (fatty acids). When we have more glucose in our body than needed, we create a toxic environment. When we lower our intake of carbohydrates and eat the adequate amounts of protein and fat, we will lose the excess body fat because the body will become efficient at burning fat for fuel, and you will not need the excessive amounts of carbohydrates.

Eating the proper amount of macronutrients daily and weekly will keep you on the right track. One of the worst things you can do is eat excess amounts of carbohydrates and fats and not get in adequate amounts of protein. So let's take a look at how to eat for optimal health expression.

Let's Not Diet

In my mind, the word "diet" is a bad word. I don't even like to say that I am dieting. It stirs feelings of deprivation in my mind. The moment I tell myself I'm dieting, it's as if a Pac-man switch is turned on, and all of a sudden I want everything I'm not supposed to have. It's funny because I don't even want this type of food when I'm not dieting. I'm convinced the word diet scrambles my brain. Like most other human beings, I do not tolerate being restricted. Saying no to something or limiting ourselves tends to make us want it more of the things we are depriving ourselves of. Silly humans.

Instead of saying that you are dieting, just say, "I'm retraining my body to become a fat-burning machine." A fat-burning machine is someone who has successfully minimized his or her carbohydrate intake to a level that works for them and then allows them to burn stored body fat as a source of fuel.

When you can limit your intake of carbohydrates to less than 150 grams per day and make up the difference with healthy fats and protein, and then add energy system training to your life, you will begin to turn your body into an efficient fat-burning machine. Becoming an effective fat burner and creating a metabolically active body is the major premise of the figureFIT! eating and exercise strategies.

You could choose a diet that is borderline ketogenic or one that is only low in carbohydrates. A ketogenic diet is when your body goes into ketosis. Ketosis is a normal metabolic process that happens when the body does not have enough carbohydrates (glucose) from food for energy for the cells, so it burns fat instead. As part of this process, it makes ketones. It impairs the glucose tolerance and the physiological insulin resistance. That sounds negative, but it is necessary to spare what little glucose exists in your body for the brain because the brain is what needs that remaining amount of glucose. A well-constructed diet of fewer carbohydrates leads to weight loss and improved insulin sensitivity.

Becoming a fat-burning machine is not something that could be or should be done in the course of one week. It takes your body time to become fat adapted. Give yourself about a month and begin to decrease the body's dependency on carbohydrates. The body will begin to burn the fat you eat, stored body fat for fuel, and will not need the excess carbohydrates. Most of the time, the struggle is in the mind because we are creatures of habit and used to eating a certain way. Give yourself some time to transition, and your body will be burning fat for fuel in no time at all.

The Difference Between a Sugar Burner and a Fat Burner

A sugar burner runs on carbohydrates. If you eat a lot of carbohydrates, there will be a constant glucose drip. When you are constantly running on carbohydrates, your body can't tap into stored fats for energy. Therefore, you will never lose weight.

To make matter worse, too many carbohydrates can make you insulin resistant over time. Insulin resistance is when your cells no longer can tell when you need to release insulin or hold on to it. That is when obesity becomes a disease because your body and cells have started to malfunction.

If you want to lose fat, you need to stop eating a lot of carbohydrates. Your body can generate the energy it needs from the fat on your body and the fat that you eat. Once the glucose is used up, hunger will set in, and you can stop the glucose cycle by reducing your carbohydrate intake and reaching for healthy proteins and fats instead.

A fat-burning machine or a fat adapted person can effectively burn fat for energy throughout the day and doesn't need the steady drip of carbohydrates. It's a huge pet peeve of mine when I hear people say, "My energy is low; I need sugar." This is the opposite of what you want to do.

When you are running off carbohydrates, your body relies on it. Then you don't burn fat easily, and you have the highs and lows to your energy throughout the day.

As you begin to lower your carbohydrate intake, eat the right amounts of protein and fats, you'll become an effective fat burner, you will be able to go hours without needing to eat, having energy dips or becoming ravenous, cranky, or craving carbohydrates. When you become a fat burner, your body can effectively oxidize dietary fat and stored body fat for fuel (energy), and this is where you want to be.

It is a process that happens slowly. But once you become fat adapted, you'll have fewer carbohydrates in your body, you'll need to keep your protein intake steady, and you'll be burning fat for fuel rather than the fat gaining short term energy source of carbohydrates - you will be less hungry and you will not have the highs and lows in mental capacity or energy because you are not getting that swing from the carbohydrates.

Ultimately, being a fat burning machine means metabolic flexibility. A fat-burning person's body will effectively burn through glucose for fuel and become efficient at turning to the fats eaten and stored for effective conversion into a usable energy source. Once you become a fat-burner, you will know how to replenish the small amount of carbs that you do need and you'll start feeling great.

There is no test you can take to find out if you are fat adapted. The easiest way to find out is to ask yourself a few basic questions:

- Can you go three hours without eating and not starve?

- Do you have steady energy throughout the day?

- Are naps a gift to yourself rather than a need or accidental thing?

- Can you exercise without eating carbohydrates before or after?

- Have the headaches and the brain fuzziness gone away?

If yes, then you are most likely fat adapted. It is the normal state of the human body.

I am currently training a client whose main goal is to have a six-pack. The other day, I asked him how he is doing, and he said, "I love that I can eat bacon and still lose weight." I agree. It is awesome when you know the right way to fuel your body.

We now know that a diet low in carbohydrates can be effective for losing body fat. However, if your intake is too low, your performance in the gym and your brain will suffer. It's best to know your macronutrient profile and hit your macros consistently.

CHAPTER 11
Macronutrients and Nutrient Timing

In this chapter, I will cover the basic elements of the figureFIT! approach to eating your macronutrients every single day at the appropriate times and why that matters.

Macronutrients

Macronutrients are protein, fats, and carbohydrates. It is important that you eat the appropriate macronutrients for your height and weight (or a weight loss macronutrient plan) every day.

The idea is that we daily eat the appropriate amount of protein and roughly fewer than 150 carbohydrates and that the rest of our macronutrients come in fat calories. Some people can eat significantly fewer carbohydrates and feel great while others, usually due to the amount of activity, may need a little more (up to 175) to satisfy their energy and cognitive function.

When you become a fat burner, you burn stored body fat for fuel, or your body uses the fat rather than the carbohydrates that you consume for fuel. Then you will notice wonderful energy and a more sustained satiety level (you won't feel hungry all the time). It is perfectly healthy to eat fewer than 50 carbohydrates per day every once in a while to allow your body to stay on the fringe of ketosis. This is called carbohydrate cycling.

As you eat this way, your body will upregulate fat burning and down-regulate fat storage. You will drop excess weight, and your body will become efficient at deriving energy from fat storages. Can you say *winning?* You can expect to lose 1 to 2 pounds per week. This is a safe fat-loss range. It is not realistic (or safe) to expect more than this weekly.

A slower rate of fat loss is much more sustainable over the long haul than extremely fast-paced fat loss. Crash diets may work for a short amount of time, but they will eventually cause the body's fight or flight response to activate. Your body will then perceive this weight loss as a starvation threat. Then the fat loss will stop, and your body will begin to store fat to preserve itself.

150 Pound Female: Kelly

Let's look at a case study of Kelly. She weighs 150 pounds, and she is 36 years old, 5 feet and 7 inches tall, and very active.

Her Needs:

1. **Basal metabolic rate:** 1,404 (calories per day)

2. **Total daily energy expenditure:** 2,054 (calories per day) Based on exercising five times per week

3. **Caloric needs for weight loss:** 1746 (calories per day) This is at a 15 percent suggested calorie reduction. Anything more than this would be considered aggressive.

Macronutrient needs:

- 150 pounds at 22 percent body fat = 108 pounds of lean body mass

- Protein: 110-135 grams per day

- Carbohydrates: 87-100 grams per day

- Fat: 97 grams per day

- Fiber: 35 grams per day

The protein needs to remain stable to maintain lean muscle mass. The variables are the fat and carbohydrates.

Breaking this down into five meals per day:

- Protein: 26.2 / meal = 131 per day

- Carbohydrates: 17.5 / meal = 87.3 per day

- Fat: 19.4 / meal = 97 per day

- Fiber: 6-8 / meal = 30-38 per day

- Total Calories: 1746

Breaking this down into six meals per day:

- Protein: 21.8 / meal = 131 per day

- Carbohydrates: 14.6 / meal = 87.3 per day

- Fat: 16.2 / meal = 97 per day

- Fiber: 5-6 / meal = 30-38 per day

- Total Calories: 1746

Nutrient Timing

It is important to understand that nutrient timing matters. You need to know what you ought to consume nutritionally before and after your workouts because feeding your muscles before and after your workout is essential. Otherwise, your body will turn to the muscles for fuel (muscle breakdown), and you will become catabolic. When you know the science behind nutrient timing, you will be better equipped to hit your fitness and weight loss goals because you will be eating to fuel your body rather than just eating anything when and where you want.

Your primary goal each day is to hit your "splits" as closely as you can. In the fitness community, we call your nutrition breakdown your splits. It is your day's macronutrients broken down into complete meals (splits) specifically consumed at specific times of the day based on your hormones and when you work out.

Since the amount of protein is the one constant, you need to make sure you hit your required protein intake every day. Remember that protein contains amino acids, which are the building blocks of every cell your body makes. If you're not consuming sufficient amounts of protein, your body will turn to muscle for those amino acids which it does when you do not fuel your body appropriately. You do not want your body to turn to your hard-earned muscle for fuel. You've worked hard for that and you want to keep it.

When building meals, it's important to put together a complete nutrient-dense meal with the proper macros. Eating snacks throughout the day will leave you nutritionally deficient and lacking vitamins and minerals that your body needs. Focus on building complete meals with the proper macro ratios.

Kelly, our example, would need to sit down and start building meals she likes that would fit the macronutrient needs that are listed below. I would recommend that each meal is a complete meal, but I understand that people have busy lives. Sometimes, a meal replacement protein shake may just have to do the trick. I consume one or two meal replacement shakes per day and often a protein-only shake at the end of the day to get in the last amounts of protein I need.

Kelly's Workout Day Splits:

Meal 1: 22 grams protein, 24 grams fat, 0 carbohydrates (vegetables are allowed)

Meal 2: 22 grams protein, 24 grams fat, 30 grams carbohydrates

(Workout) - perhaps add 30 grams of carbohydrates during her workout and lower the carbohydrates at each meal before and after the workout.

Meal 3: 22 grams protein, 0 fat, 30 grams carbohydrates

Meal 4: 22 grams protein, 0 fat, 27 grams carbohydrates

Meal 5: 22 grams protein, 24 grams fat, 0 carbohydrates (vegetables are allowed)

Meal 6: 22 grams protein, 24 grams fat, 0 carbohydrates (vegetables are allowed)

In this model of nutrient timing, you can see that the protein remains steady throughout the day. We then focus our carbohydrates before and after our workouts to refuel the body's lost glycogen. The rest of the day, we fill in the macros with healthy fats from avocados, nuts, seeds, and high-quality oils with no carbohydrates (unless it's vegetables).

The numbers listed here are an example and may be changed based on the client's goals and needs. Maybe she wants to gain more muscle. If that is the case, we would need to tweak her calories and add calories to her diet. To accomplish your physique changing goals, you should eat the exact amount of fat, carbohydrates, protein, and fiber listed in your macro splits every day, regardless of whether or not you exercise.

Please remember that these numbers are a guide and specific to our example above. The macronutrient way of eating can't account for metabolism damage or poor health, so some modifications may need to be made in those cases.

Most of my clients see changes after only four weeks of eating this way. In some cases, when no changes are seen, my clients are consuming too many calories – or too few in some rare occasions (or when working out more than suggested). In those cases, we work with clients to adjust accordingly. We only make minor changes by manipulating the amount of carbohydrates by no more than 10 grams per week until we see the scale move, or the client sees physical changes in their body. There is no need to reduce carbohydrates by more than 10 grams per week or make major moves in calorie restriction when you're seeing results.

Also, there is no reason to change your macros if you are still losing weight! We keep on keeping on when something is working and tweak it when needed for changes in muscle gain or weight loss.

CHAPTER 12
Lifestyle Tools and Supplements

We often hear about different supplements that will help us burn fat, improve our metabolism, sleep better, etc. The fact is our bodies are made to function properly when we are taking care of it. We don't need much other than good foods, quality sleep, and water to keep the body running at an optimal level. So save your money on all so-called quick fixes that don't work, live life according to the figureFIT! lifestyle, and implement the tools below instead.

Your Body's Best Supplement: High-Quality Protein

Consumption of protein is so important that I ask the following question on the final exam of my yoga teacher training program: "What is the importance of protein in the human diet?" As part of my program, I teach my trainees about nutrition science. It is essential that people understand the basic principles of nutrition science and how our bodies utilize protein, fats, and carbohydrates. This information should be taught in all schools and built upon over the years. But the sad fact is that it is not taught in schools. Not even physicians are taught about nutrition science or gut health. Whenever I get a chance to teach about proper nutrition, I do because it is the foundation for health. Medicine is not. If nutrition science and gut health were taught in schools, our society would look very different. Fewer people would be overweight, and fewer people would be sick.

When I ask my yoga students the question about the importance of protein on their final exam, I often get a variety of answers. They say, for example:

"Protein is for muscle building."

"Protein makes you stronger."

"Protein has amino acids that build muscles."

We have a tendency to think that protein shakes are only for people who are trying to build muscle such as bodybuilders. People see bodybuilders drinking protein shakes, and they are so warped by the bodybuilding industry that they think only bodybuilders need to supplement with protein.

The fact is that we all need protein. As I have said before, protein contains amino acids that are the building blocks of every new cell in your body. I explain it like this to my teacher trainee students: The amino acids in protein are the frame to the cells your body is trying to make. Just like if you were to build a house, you would want a strong foundation and sturdy walls. That is what the protein will do for your cells. If you don't eat protein, only carbohydrates and fats, your body is building weak and deformed cells that will not last long.

High-quality protein is the primary supplement to add to your daily nutrition if you want to prevent muscle breakdown, build strong and healthy cells, drop body fat, and enhance your overall health.

Loss of muscle in the human body is called sarcopenia. It is a condition that impacts each and every one of us. Our muscle mass peaks when we are around 30 years old. From that age going forward, adults start to lose approximately 0.5 pound of muscle and gain 1 pound of fat per year. That is if you're not working out and focusing your meals around a good-quality protein.

The human body evolved through times of intermittent fasting, and it will ultimately store a little bit of fat as a reserve for emergency supplies when food is scarce. Any excess fat, however, will hinder your body's optimal functioning. Fat gain that exceeds our body's normal fat reserves will begin to build up around vital internal organs causing major problems. This type of fat is called "visceral fat," which lies deep within the body and poses a great risk to our health.

According to Ronenn Roubenoff and Carmen Castaneda, "sarcopenia is the backdrop against which the drama of disease is played out."[23] If you're not getting enough protein, your body can't fight illness or degeneration. Even if your body weight is normal, having a high percentage of body fat puts you at an increased risk for chronic disease.

Maintaining our muscle mass is important for our overall health and the development of new cells. It also helps us to prevent buildup of bad fat around our internal organs. When we maintain our muscle mass, we keep our metabolism higher, support our joints, boost our immunity, and keep our heart healthier.

The biggest problem my clients usually have when they are reaching for their goals is they are not eating their body's daily allotment of protein. The second biggest problem is they're not staying consistent with the workouts. That's it. If they would stick to these two things, everything else would eventually fall into place as long as they are not abusing other substances like sugar, fat, and alcohol, and they are getting enough sleep.

A good quality protein is instrumental in maintaining a healthy lifestyle, but not all proteins are created equal. I recommend whey and casein to my clients. Real food is the foundation for a healthy diet. However, whey protein is much more than a muscle-builder and meal replacer. I would argue that it is just as important as brushing your teeth.

---

[23] Roubenoff, R., & Castaneda, C. (2001, September 12). Sarcopenia-Understanding the Dynamics of Aging Muscle. Retrieved August 12, 2015, from http://jama.jamanetwork.com/article.aspx?articleid=194167

When it comes to dairy, the issue of tolerance arises. Many people cannot tolerate dairy whether it's the lactose or the proteins. As Mark Sisson points out, "most people can tolerate whey without issue. You're far more likely to be allergic, sensitive, or intolerant to lactose or casein than to whey."[24] Just because you have a problem with milk or yogurts, don't count out a high-quality whey supplement. Whey protein formulas have shown to be effective in the prevention of many allergic diseases such as asthma and eczema in susceptible children and infants.[25]

Whey protein isolates or whey protein hydrolysis are the best forms of protein blends. They are a higher quality and contain more protein than other forms of protein powder blends. They also have fewer carbohydrates and fat, and they are perfect for pre- and post-workout since they're digested and absorbed quickly.

Whey protein is digested quickly, which makes it a fantastic post-workout fuel to help build and repair the muscles you just worked. The moment you ingest a protein shake, the amino acids break down rapidly and are absorbed into the bloodstream. Your blood then escorts the amino acids to the muscle tissues you just worked to help with protein synthesis.

Whey protein also boosts blood flow to muscle tissue, which is another secret of its protein synthesis power. Increased blood flow enhances the delivery of nutrients, including glucose (energy), amino acids, and oxygen. These nutrients support muscle growth and spur recovery after a workout. This is the primary reason I recommend protein supplement shakes to my clients.

---

[24] The Health Benefits of Whey Protein | Mark's Daily Apple. (2014, November 26). Retrieved August 12, 2015, from http://www.marksdailyapple.com/not-just-for-bodybuilders-the-many-wheys-whey-protein-can-improve-your-health/#axzz3ie7MM1EG

[25] Clin, J. (2002, August 1). Food hypersensitivity and allergic diseases. Retrieved August 12, 2015, from http://www.ncbi.nlm.nih. gov/pubmed/12142964

When to Take Whey Supplements

Due to the fast absorption rate, the two most critical times to consume your whey protein or meal replacement shakes are 15 to 30 minutes before your workouts and within 30 minutes after your workouts.

Providing your body with quickly digested amino acids before, during, and immediately after your figureFIT! workouts promotes maximal muscle growth. When you consume whole-food protein sources like chicken breast, eggs, fish, and beef, it is not digested fast enough to be beneficial for muscle repair.

Before weight training, take about [15-18] grams of whey protein to enhance muscle strength, increase endurance, and decrease muscle breakdown. After your workouts, go with 20-40 grams of whey to enhance muscle recovery and boost muscle protein synthesis.

You should also consider taking 20-40 grams of whey protein as soon as you roll out of bed. This will stop the muscle breakdown that occurs as a result of fasting overnight. You can also drink a 20-40 gram whey shake as a snack between meals to boost muscle growth and support fat loss.[26]

The Importance of Water

Water makes up 60 percent of your body weight and is essential to a host of bodily functions, including carrying nutrients to your cells and creating a moist environment for nose, ear and throat tissues. Since your body neither makes nor stores water, drinking fluids every day is necessary to restore what you lose through sweat and urination. Cool water is the best fluid for hydration during and after workouts.

[26] Stoppani, J. (2015, March 19). Whey To Transform: Your Expert Guide To The Premier Muscle-Building Protein - Bodybuilding. com. Retrieved August 12, 2015, from http://www.bodybuilding. com/fun/whey-to-grow-expert-guide-premier-muscle-building-protein. html

Everyone should drink at least 8 cups daily, although athletes need more.[27]

I recommend that you have one ounce of water for every pound that you weigh. Do the math and make it happen. In the beginning, you will be going to the bathroom quite a bit, but after a couple of days, your body will adjust, and you'll get into a more regular pattern. We have to remember that our body is 50 to 65 percent water, and we need water to assist every vital function in our body. Here are some top reasons to sip water throughout the day:

Water can help to boost your metabolism. Drink a full liter of cold water first thing in the morning to fire up your metabolism. When we wake up, the body temperature is higher, so consuming cold water will put your body to work. Your body will then go to work heating the water to your body's temperature. I find that after about ten minutes of drinking the cold water, I start to feel more awake, the hunger pangs that I may have had are gone, and I feel refreshed.

Water helps to maintain the balance of body fluids.

Your body is composed or 60% water. The functions of these bodily fluids include digestion, absorption, circulation, creation of saliva, transportation of nutrients, and maintenance of body temperature. The brain communicates with the kidneys and tells it how much water to excrete as urine or hold onto for reserves. When you are low on fluids, the brain triggers the body's thirst mechanism.[28]

NOTE: Alcohol is not a good choice for a beverage. "Alcohol interferes with the brain and kidney communication and causes excess excretion of fluids, which can lead to dehydration.[29]"

---

[27] Lewis, R. (2014, March 13). Does Drinking Cold Water Help Speed Up Your Metabolism? Retrieved August 12, 2015, from http:// www. livestrong.com/article/521032-does-drinking-cold-water-help-speed-up-your-metabolism/

[28] Stark, A. (2011, July 3). Dehydration Essay. Retrieved August 12, 2015, from http://www.antiessays.com/free-essays/Dehydration-165486.html

[29] Zelman, K. (2008, May 8). Why Drink More Water? See 6 Health Benefits of Water. Retrieved August 12, 2015, from http://www.webmd.com /diet/6-reasons-to-drink-water?page=1

Water helps to control calories. Often when you think you're hungry, you're actually thirsty. If you are adequately hydrated, you are not going to have a tendency to overeat. Although drinking water cannot make you lose weight, dieters have been using this strategy for years because you keep yourself full.

Water helps to energize muscles. Muscle cells need adequate amounts of water to function properly. If you begin to dehydrate, your muscles will not work as well, and your performance can suffer. Drinking enough fluids is important when exercising. I follow the American College of Sports Medicine guidelines for fluid intake before and during physical activity: 17 ounces of fluid about two hours before exercise and continuously throughout to replace fluids lost by sweating.

Water keeps skin looking good. The key to beautiful skin is to keep yourself hydrated and avoid skin irritating products and foods (such as diary). "Your skin contains plenty of water, and functions as a protective barrier to prevent excess fluid loss."[30] Dehydrated skin can increase the appearance of wrinkles. Do not worry about drinking too much water because your body will only hold on to what it needs. The kidneys will excrete all excess water. After you shower, you can help "lock" moisture into your skin by using a full-body skin moisturizer and face lotion, which creates a physical barrier that keeps in the moisture.

Water helps your kidneys do their job.

Your kidneys do an amazing job of cleansing and ridding your body of toxins as long as your intake of fluids is adequate. When you get enough fluids, urine is light in color and free of odor.[30]

Water helps to maintain proper bowel function.

Adequate hydration keeps things flowing along your gastrointestinal tract and prevents constipation. When you do not get enough fluid,

---

[30] Zelman, K. (2008, May 8). Why Drink More Water? See 6 Health Benefits of Water. Retrieved August 12, 2015, from http://www. webmd.com /diet/6-reasons-to-drink-water?page=1

the colon pulls water from stools to maintain hydration, and the result is constipation.

Constipation is a very big problem with people eating the SAD (standard American diet). Many people have constipation issues for reasons we discussed in Chapter 8.

Often when I read through my client intake forms, I see people drinking on average between three to five glasses of water per day. The first thing I tell them is that their water intake needs increase drastically. Many of their health concerns can be solved simply by adding more water to their diet. So when you think you are hungry or tired, have a big glass of water first.

A Word on Caffeine

Most people consume caffeine wrong. They think, "I'm going to have a cup of coffee, and it will give me energy and fuel my workout." However, coffee is not helpful for your workout because of the acid it contains.

Caffeine itself is beneficial, but it is important to get it from the right source. Studies have been done on the results of caffeine from different sources before a workout. They have found that caffeine from green tea and caffeine supplement is better than caffeine from coffee.

Caffeine can increase performance, and it can increase fat for fuel during post-exercise. But if you make the wrong choice in caffeine, the caffeine will work against you because of some of the hormones it influences.

Dr. Terry Graham is one of the world's foremost caffeine researchers. He performed a study where one group received pure caffeine, and the other group received caffeine from coffee. The group that got pure caffeine had the expected improvement in exercise performance, but the group that had coffee did not. It appeared that one or more of the chemicals or nutrients in coffee impaired the positive effects of the caffeine.

Caffeine seems to enhance all the major alterations of the body to prepare itself for exercise. It boosts levels of adrenaline, and it lowers adenosine. Adrenaline also inhibits the hormone insulin and increases levels of glucagon. This combination signalizes the body to flood the blood with glucose, which provides the muscles with energy to contract and move helping you to get in a great workout.

PART 3

figure*FIT!*

FITNESS

CHAPTER 13
figure*FIT!* Workouts:
Energy System Training

Science of Maximal Fat Burning and Boosted Metabolism

Training fads come and go in bodybuilding and fitness, and there have been thousands of them over the decades. Some appear, disappear, and then get rehashed a few years later under a different name. Only a small number catch on and become a must for people who want serious results, and those are the ones that are backed by science.

Anybody who knows anything about getting an excellent physique knows that lifting weights is a must. It is the first step because you *need* muscles to move the body. Muscle is metabolically active, which means that it is *hungry!* A person with muscle will have a higher metabolism that someone without muscle.

When it comes to fat burning, the following three components take the cake!

1. Building muscle with a strength training program

2. Becoming a fat-burning machine by incorporating the figureFIT! Nutrition Program.

3. Doing high-intensity interval training via the figureFIT! workouts.

High-intensity interval training is the best way to burn the most amount of fat in the shortest amount of time, and it will take your fat burning to a whole new level.

Many people believe that a steady state cardio, such as jogging, spinning, or some other mindless activity, is the best way to exercise. However, science has proven this to be wrong. To train effectively, lose weight, boost your metabolism, and be smart with your body's energy systems, it's important that you understand the ramifications of what your cardio and training style does to your body.

If you are truly interested in getting the best body, lose the most amount of fat, and boost your metabolism, why would you spend your time doing things that are not in your best interest? I know many people who have an old school dogmatic mindset that hours of running, spinning, and jogging are going to do the trick, yet they are the ones who remain overweight. This strategy may have worked for them once or twice in their life, so it becomes their go-to strategy from that day out. But when something is not working for you - it is not working for you and doing something different is required. I see it all of the time, I ask people what they like to do and they answer: run, walk, jog, spinning, all cardio exercises. But the fact is, chronic cardio is not smart training because it's not training the body's energy systems.

So what is the best way to train?

First off you need to focus on strength so weight lifting is essential. You need muscles to move your body. If you don't have muscles your bones and joints will weaken quicker. In addition, muscles are a metabolically active, which means they consume many of the calories you take in. The more muscle you have, the more calories you burn. However, outside of wanting a strong athletic body, the best reason to lift weights is to keep your bones strong and prevent osteoporosis - this alone is reason enough to lift weights a couple of days per week for your entire life.

Second, the high-intensity interval training (HIIT) philosophy is well accepted among the best trainers, coaches, and sports scientists. It is now considered a core training strategy for the most serious physique athletes as well as those who just want to burn body fat. The simple fact is that if you are not doing high-intensity interval training, you are missing out on the single most effective means of torching body fat and improving your overall fitness level in the shortest amount of time possible.

I have taken the science of energy system training and muscle building and turned it into workouts that you can do at home or the gym. The figureFIT! workouts incorporate both methods in one workout, so you get the best bang for your time. The members of the figureFIT! community receive three workouts per month, and they do each of the three each week. They can, for example, do Workout #1 on Monday, Workout #2 on Wednesday, and Workout #3 on Friday. Some clients of mine who were new to exercising started with one session per week and slowly added the other workouts, as they got stronger and faster. The key is just to get started wherever you are, build on as you go, and never stop or quit. As long as you're doing something, remember that is always better than nothing. The moment you quit - you're quitting on yourself, so show up every day and put in time on those workouts. As a trainer, I'm going to tell you to track your numbers and weights. Always be trying to do better today than yesterday and when you do that, even if it's only by one, you gain in strength and power, oh and above all confidence and self-love.

Let's take a moment to explore high-intensity interval training or HIIT. HIIT is made up of sessions in which you combine high levels of intense activity with lower levels of lower intensity cardio or recovery. This takes your exercise session a step beyond increasing the overall calories you burn. It allows you to recover during your slower bouts so that you can physically and (most importantly, in my opinion) mentally push harder during the intense part of your exercise. This type of training provides the most dramatic results in fat and calorie burning seen in sports science research to date. Research findings show that clients continue to burn more calories and fat after they have finished the high-intensity exercise. Yes, the workouts are tough, but you will continue to burn calories for longer periods of time (up to 32 hours) after your workouts are completed.

This type of training differs from steady state cardio in a very dramatic way. When you are running, spinning, or walking, your body is in an aerobic energy state (burning oxygen). In this state, you're not building muscle – you're not tapping into your anaerobic energy system. When you remain in this phase, you burn calories, but you're not doing anything for your future self. When you train the figureFIT! way, you increase muscle and train the body's anaerobic energy system. By doing both of these things, you increase your body's metabolism *after* the workout is over. Let's take a look at how this works.

The Body's Energy Conversion System

To understand how to raise your metabolism, you need to know about the body's three energy systems.

Introducing the powerful three / energy systems timeline. Let us say that you head outside for a sprint, and you want to see how fast and hard you can run before you start tuckering out. Here is what happens:

0 to 10 seconds: the ATP-CP system. The moment you start sprinting, all three energy systems begin to work, but the first to fire up is the ATP-CP (or phosphagen) system. This is the stored ATP within the working muscles. There is not much of this compound, so we burn through it in less than 10 seconds.

10 to 75 seconds: the glycolytic system (anaerobic system). Once ATP-CP has started to run out, the glycolytic system ramps up and takes over for the next minute or so before it too begins to run out of fuel. Glycolysis relies on energy converted from stored carbohydrates (glucose) into ATP.

75 seconds to 10 or more minutes: the oxidative system (aerobic system). The oxidative system has been generating energy the entire time the first two systems are at work, but it is also busy fueling other bodily projects such as cardiovascular function, digestion, and toxin elimination via sweat. The oxidative system uses fat as its primary fuel, but since fat takes longer to convert to energy than glucose, you will be compelled to slow down. Once this system kicks in, it can stay on the job for quite a while if you are well trained.

All three metabolic energy systems are switched on during physical activity, but each one plays a different role depending on the activity and its demands. All three systems affect metabolism, fat loss, and muscle building efforts. Let us take a closer look at these three amazing systems and how they work.

First responder: the ATP-CP system. The first responder is the adenosine triphosphate creatine phosphate (ATP-CP) system or phosphagen system. There is a small amount of ATP stored away in our muscles that is ready for fast and quick movements. This system is the fueled by our muscles, and it is the first, yet very brief, source of energy. The ATP system is the most prepared for emergencies or fast, explosive movements. It kicks in when the body's normal oxidative system is not prepared for the task.

We use the ATP system, for example, when we do a max weight squat or a single burpee, when we jump up to get the phone, or when we quickly reach to stop a vase from falling. The energy of this system lasts for less than 10 seconds.

All three energy systems ultimately run on ATP; it is the fuel source for all physical functions, from breathing to sprinting up a hill. Your other two systems (glycolytic and oxidative) make ATP when they are waiting to be used.

Next up: the glycolytic energy system. The second system we tap into is the glycolytic system. This system is fueled by glycogen (stored carbohydrates or sugar). It provides energy for activities of slightly longer duration such as strength training and high intense intervals.

Training the glycolytic system will strengthen all three systems and help them work together more efficiently. In addition, you will burn more fat in the long run because the recovery period from training this system requires work from all three energy systems. After a workout that trains the glycolytic system, your body is ramped up due to EPOC (which we will discuss in a moment) and burning stored body fat for fuel up to 48 hours after the workout simply trying to help you recover. Can you say figureFIT? This is the power of the figureFIT! workouts.

If you have ever tried to sprint the entire way around a track, you are aware of what it feels like to exercise the glycolytic system; it is tough! However, the discomfort and effort that comes from training the glycolytic system is well worth it because if you want to lose fat, gain muscle, and get the most out of your precious gym time, this is the system to train.

Last and long burning: the oxidative system. The third system we tap into is the oxidative system. This system is fueled by fat and glucose, but it is the only system that requires oxygen to function. The oxidative system is always at work and is the system that sustains all of our bodies' functions. Although the oxidative system is continuously active, the process of converting fat into usable energy can take a while. Once it gets started, though, it is your body's most sustained source over long periods of time.

Exercise physiologists used to believe that long, slow cardio exercises practiced for an hour or more several times a week was the best way to train this system. But research has proven that the oxidative system works very hard to help you recover after anaerobic (glycolytic) training. Unless you are a competitive endurance athlete, loads of long slow cardio is probably not the best way to train your aerobic system. Through high-intensity training, you can significantly increase the capacity of your aerobic system and burn more fat.

How to Train Your Energy Systems for Maximal Metabolic Functioning

Training your ATP-CP system and glycolytic systems (anaerobic training). I create three workouts per month for the participants of my program. If you follow the program, you will do each workout one time per week. Each workout focuses on combination body moves that will incorporate your core muscles and other muscles of the body. For example: In Workout #1, we may do eight exercises. We will focus on doing three exercises in a row without stopping. We will then take a short break up to two to three minutes to catch our breath and recover and then we will repeat the exercise three to four more times. Then we move on to the next set of exercises and follow in the same sequence. This type of training works the body's ATP-CP and glycolytic systems - this is anaerobic training. When we stop to rest, the body's oxidative (aerobic) system kicks in to help us recover and continues for up to 36-48 hours post workout.

People who train the ATP-CP system are fast, strong and explosive and will have amazing results in single-effort activities. We train this system with sprinting, maximum efforts, and short and intense bouts of exercise. Training the ATP-CP energy system will not increase the stores of ATP-CP in the muscles (because that is fixed in the body), but it will improve your explosive speed and power. As a result, you can jump higher, sprint faster, and throw further. Training this system is the best way to increase your power and speed.

We train the ATP-CP and glycolytic systems in the figureFIT! workouts. Our work period lasts between 30 seconds and two minutes or so. Athletes who train this way become fast, recover more quickly, and tend to be muscular and lean. This is one of the best ways to train for fat burning and muscle building.

Training your oxidative system. We train our oxidative system when we jog, run long-distance, cycle, use traditional cardio machines, or slow swimming.

Although it is last to kick in, the oxidative system is always working in the background. One could say it is the most important energy system of all because it is what keeps your body operating. It is always running in the background keeping every system operating via oxygen. Oxidative athletes are typically leaner and lighter than the other two athletic types. They can go on forever at a slow-to-medium pace, burning mostly fat, which is the ultimate high-efficiency, slow-burning fuel. Oxidative training is essential for endurance sports, but all athletes should train this system. Done in moderation, oxidative training is also great for helping you recover from other, more intense forms of exercise.

Training all three systems is extremely important. But it has been proven that training the first two systems will automatically strengthen the third (oxidative) system, meaning it is highly at work when you are recovering from those high intense training sessions. There are numerous studies showing that people who only train their oxidative system with long bouts of cardio are harming their body, especially if they are not taking in enough calories or are overloaded with stress.

So do yourself a favor, strengthen the first two energy systems by shortening the length of your gyms session, upping the weight and intensity, and go hard for a shorter time with max effort intensity. Your body will thank you.

Make it easy for yourself by signing up for the figureFIT! Lifestyle Program and let me plan your workout for you. As I said, every month, I create three different workouts that you will do over the course of the month. These workouts incorporate all the different techniques listed above. They are tough, but over the course of the month, you will build up to doing the entire workout. Beginners start out the program either by doing the moves without weights or only one time through or both. Advanced athletes simply add more weight to make the workouts tougher. They can also add sets to the workouts.

It's important to train at your level and give yourself time to increase your metabolic capacity. Don't overdo it. I help all our members with their training goals. We will set a goal to train each system at least once per week in the beginning. Then we increase your training sessions each week until you are at a max training schedule for your body and goals. The body is incredible and will respond very fast to this type of training regimen.

Understanding the Post Exercise Results – Oxidative Max and EPOC

When the body has enough oxygen (aerobic energy), it will use the aerobic energy pathway. But when the oxygen supplies run out, the body switches to an anaerobic pathway. To get into an anaerobic training zone, you have to work quite hard. The idea of high-intensity interval training is that you work in an anaerobic training zone, which helps to boost your resting metabolic rate. Doing that also increases something scientists call EPOC, which is excess post-exercise oxygen consumption.

EPOC is the result of the body doing more *after* you have finished working out to help your body recover. That is a good thing, and it requires calories. This type of training also increases your VO2 max, which is the maximum amount of oxygen your body can use during exercise.

VO2 max is a measure of the maximum volume of oxygen that someone can use. It measures how much oxygen your lungs can take in, convert into the blood stream, and pump through your body by your heart. It also measures how efficiently your muscles consume and convert that oxygen for use. Since oxygen is the most critical component in operating at a higher intensity, your VO2 max is the best measure of your fitness level. As you begin with the figureFIT! workouts, your VO2 rate will increase. It will continue to do so until you have reached the point where you can no longer utilize oxygen any faster. That is your VO2 max.

A good example of this is my long-time client Anne McConville. Anne is in her 50's, she's a long-time marathon runner and was consistently held out at a pace of 3:49. After adding in the figureFIT! workouts, Anne took 10 minutes off her time. Simply put, her body got better and better at recovery and she could go harder and faster. By training her anaerobic system for this first time in decades, she gained a better VO2 max and her fitness level increased making her faster.

The higher your VO2 max, the better your fitness level is. We all want a higher VO2 max because this means that the body can process more calories and oxygen, which can increase performance in any given time frame.

At the peak of your high-intensity interval, when you create an oxygen debt, your body has burned off all the available blood sugar and starts to burn more fat for energy. You don't want your body to use fat as an energy source during exercise because fat takes longer to convert to ATP. But after your training is over, burning fat is ideal. This is why we consume a specific amount high-quality carbohydrates (along with our other macros) before and after workouts.

Back in 1996, Professor Izumi Tabata studied the effects of moderate intensity endurance versus high-intensity intermittent training on anaerobic capacity and VO2 max at the National Institute of Fitness and Sports in Japan. The study concluded that adequate high-intensity intermittent training may improve both anaerobic and aerobic energy supply systems significantly, and the rate of improvement in VO2 max was one of the highest ever reported.

The world's most highly respected sports scientist at McMaster University also performed a study on high-intensity interval training. In the study, they used a high-intensity interval training protocol, which included 60 seconds of intense exercise at 95 percent VO2 max, followed by 75 seconds of rest repeated for 8 to 12 cycles. The results showed that from *just three sessions per week,* the effect of this training was comparable to training five hours per week at a 50 to 70 percent VO2 max.

American College of Sports Medicine found that with just four to six 30-second sprints with 4-minute low-intensity intervals in between resulted in body fat losses of *over 12 percent* in six weeks. The group that exercised twice as long by doing traditional running lost less than 6 percent body fat.

The figureFIT! workouts are high-intensity intervals and the single most effective method to burn fat. Going back to Anne, my client who took 10 minutes off her marathon after doing the figureFIT! workouts for a year. Ten minutes is *huge* to a marathon runner. High-intensity interval training is used more and more as the most effective way to increase endurance and improve the athletic performance of top athletes, Olympians, and sports teams. It is not just for elite athletes. For peak health and fitness, everybody should train this way. I created this program so that I can take you from where you are to where you want to be by training your energy systems in this manner. All you have to do is start.

On the figureFIT! Lifestyle Program, we do the following:

1. We understand *who* we are and re-remember that daily via meditation and prayer.

2. We eat for optimal health and understand what the foods we are eating do to our bodies.

3. We train our bodies' energy systems to maximal workout effectiveness.

4. We stay connected to our tribe to give and receive support, love, and encouragement.

CHAPTER 14
Yoga, It's Much More Than People Realize

I struggled as to where to put this chapter in this book because yoga is tremendous for helping you uncover your true happiness, so I wanted to include it in Part 1: Happy = Mindset, or in chapter 5 Stress; because yoga is probably one of the best things you can do to de-stress. I decided to include it here in the end under Part 3 = FITNESS because what people tend to think of when they see or hear yoga is the physical poses. I include it here in the figureFIT! section, simply because of the physical aspect of the practice that most people see but it's time you learn what yoga truly is.

Yoga is much more than what we see; it's a way of life. When someone heads to their first yoga class, they don't know that they just tipped over the first domino in a succession that will teach them about who they are. That is if they continue down this path of self-discovery.

The path of yoga is about living an ethical life and having a clean body. It is also about letting go of attachments that hold you back, focusing the mind, and aligning yourself with the divinity that lives within. It is a daily practice that goes far beyond the yoga poses. The poses, called asanas, are tools to help you focus the mind. They are tools that lead you to the deeper parts of yourself. This self is often called the observer. It's the part of us that is unchangeable, divine, perfect, and all-knowing, and it lives within each and every one of us.

The yoga poses help the body, yes, but it's more than that. The practice of asana (the poses) combines deep breathing and movement and this has an amazing effect it has on the body's central nervous system and how it calms the mind. The practice of yoga encompasses the connection between the mind and body, and it helps both. It helps the digestive, cardiovascular, lymph, and all other systems of the body. Yoga is a magic elixir that helps to heal you physically and mentally. But like I said before, yoga goes beyond the poses, it's truly a way of life that you only discover once you tip that first domino.

A Personal Journey

After I graduated college in 2000, I bought a yoga DVD. This simple little act was the first domino to many lives that would eventually be healed and jobs created via what came of my personal yoga journey. The DVD had an AM yoga sequence, a PM yoga sequence, and a more advanced yoga sequence. I started doing the AM yoga sequence before work. I realized that this gentle morning practice woke up my body, made me feel good, and gave my mind a sense of calm and clarity. I felt that this practice connected me to my inner Holy Spirit. I would feel wonderful after the gentle morning session, and I would take this sense of peace with me into my day and infuse this laid-back attitude into everything I did. On the days I didn't do the yoga, on the other hand, I felt stress from the day.

A couple of years later, I went to a yoga class and had an awakening as to what a hard yoga class was all about. The class that I went to was for advanced yogis, and I was anything but that. I found myself in positions that were extremely challenging to hold, and I was cussing out the yoga teacher in my head thinking, "What the heck is her problem? Is she trying to kill me?" I had no idea what I gotten myself into by joining this particular class, and I didn't enjoy it at all. I thought that I would be going to a class that was similar to what I used to practice in the mornings before work. However, the poses that I found myself trying to do were immensely difficult, and my body was not ready for this type of practice. I left that class never wanting to go to another.

Another few years down the road, I went to a yoga class in Santa Monica, California. This was when I realized that yoga could be both a gentle practice and advanced practice for skilled athletes. This class was spiritually based, and it was an intermediate level class. The room was candlelit, and the teacher was studying psychology, so she intertwined psychology through the entire yoga practice.

I am a deeply spiritual person, and when the teacher connected the spiritual part of the yoga path to the physical practice, I fell in love with it. The class was physically challenging, but at the end of the class, when I was in the last pose called Savasana, tears streamed down my face. The spiritual aspect intertwined with the practice made me feel cracked wide open yet very hopeful about my future. I saw life and yoga differently, and I felt different.

After the class, as I was walking down the street with my friend, I had a light feeling about me. It felt as if I was floating between each step. I asked my friend, "What the heck has happened to me? I feel like I'm floating." My friend said, "Oh, you have the yoga high." I had no idea what *that* was, but I knew I needed to find out more about this amazing practice. I didn't drink or smoke anything to feel this way, all I did was practice yoga in a dark room and breathe deeply for an hour. I knew I needed whatever had just happened to me, and I needed this on a daily basis.

On my way home from California that weekend, I stopped at a bookstore and got three magazines: *Yoga Journal, Oxygen Magazine,* and *Entrepreneur Magazine.* I was so inspired that I set some goals for myself on the airplane that day. My first goal was to become a yoga teacher so that I could learn more about this powerful practice. My second goal was to enter a fitness competition. My third goal was to open my own business.

To become a yoga teacher, I enrolled in a local school called Green Tree School of Yoga. The yoga scene in my town was pretty small, and if you were to find a yoga class, chances were it was in someone's home or basement. I wasn't interested in that as that seemed a bit creepy to me.

Then it hit me; my town needed a large and mainstream yoga studio. I started doing some planning and research, and I became confident that this was the business to go for. I had a full-time job, but opening a yoga studio was now my dream, so I worked on it on the side. I began developing a business plan and creating the content for the website.

That same year, I entered my first and only fitness competition. Within the year, I had completed two of my goals, and I had taken steps towards the third, which was opening my own business.

In 2009, I became a yoga teacher, and in 2010, I finalized the details, the content, and the planning for the yoga studio. In January 2011, I opened Solace Yoga Studio.

The reason I share this with you is that it goes back to the vision board we discussed in Chapter 4: "Set Yourself Up to Win." Create big goals for yourself and start going after them one day at a time. It's just like this lifestyle program; success will only come to those who put in place the tools and live this lifestyle on a consistent basis. When you create a plan, only you can stop yourself from achieving your goals by not staying focused. I hope that has become clear by now.

The reason I have been able to achieve what I have in life is because I go after what I want. My daily practice of pushing myself to think better and bigger thoughts, work harder in the gym, and eat the right foods has opened up my life up in many ways both personally and professionally. Why are so many successful entrepreneurs fit? It's because they know the value of a healthy body and mind, so they incorporate healthy practices into their daily life.

Owning a yoga studio has been an amazing blessing, and it has also been very challenging. The beauty of the yoga practice comes in the entire path of yoga. It's far more than the poses that you see in Instagram photos. Yoga is a path to enlightenment. It helps you in all areas of your life. The first class you take (that you enjoy) is like the first domino in a series of events that end up changing you and shaping your life. I can say this because I've seen it first hand with thousands of people who come through the doors of my yoga studio. Clients will call me, email me, or post on social media and tell me how their yoga practice changed their life. I'm still in awe sometimes that this life I created through my entrepreneurial spirit and natural desire to bring peace to people has helped so many. I literally shine from the inside out when someone is touched by yoga - when they see the true benefits of it.

Yoga begins to undo the crazy that you (or life) has placed onto you over the years. You become more in tune with your true inner self, your habits, your ego, and you slowly begin to shed all the layers that do not serve you or your life. Through yoga comes self-awareness and this self-awareness begins to reveal the bad habits, negative beliefs, ego patterns, and negative ways you have treated yourself (and others) over the years, and more. I like to say yoga helps you to become more you. You tap into that still small voice within and THAT is the voice you need to be listening to, not your ego.

In the ancient text of The Yoga Sutras of Patanjali there are 200 sutras (like a scripture) and in those 200 sutras, yoga is explained. But in all actuality, in 2nd sutra out of 200 is the entire goal of yoga explained in that one sutra: "The restraint of the modifications of mind-stuff is Yoga." The book goes on to explain in the rest of the 198 sutras how we are to go about doing this one thing. How do we still the fluctuations of the mind? "If you can control the rising of the mind into ripples, you will experience Yoga." Yoga means union (or yoke). Union with what? The divine of course. We're all divine, remember me telling you that earlier in the introduction? Well it comes back to this. This book is yoga. Yoga in another way. Yoga is anything that helps you to still the fluctuations of the mind. If you fixing your health helps your mind - you're doing yoga. If your workout helps to clear your mind - you're doing yoga. If your playtime with your child helps you to clear your mind - you're doing yoga. Yoga is union with the divine and it comes in many ways.

Opening a yoga studio in my town in the Midwest was challenging because here we have many conservative Catholics and Christians who view yoga as Hinduism. What they fail to understand is that yoga is older than Hinduism, Buddhism, and Christianity. They also fail to understand is that yoga is *not* a religion. Yoga has been taken up as a practice by people of all religions.

Yoga is a way of living that promotes an ethical life. It can help you understand your mental afflictions (problems and attachments), take care of your body, and practice a good form of exercise. It also clears and focuses your mind, and it helps you get rid of attachments and de-stress. Yoga helps you merge with what you can call the Universal Spirit, God, or simply energy, whatever feels right to you. The fact of the matter is that yoga is a beautiful practice, and it is scientifically proven that it can benefit you in many ways.

Yoga, Deep Breathing, and GABA = Your Stress Relieving Elixir

After I had become a yoga teacher, I learned what it was was that had given me that floating sensation that one day after I left that magical yoga class in Santa Monica. It was the release of GABA, also known as gamma-aminobutyric acid. This is a natural neurotransmitter in the body that calms the central nervous system.[31] It is released in higher amounts in a yoga practice than in other documented forms of exercise.

Boston University did a study where they compared a group of yoga practitioners with a group of walkers.[32] They found that those who did yoga had a higher release of GABA than those who went for walks.

We've all heard that walking is great for our health, and I wouldn't disagree. Some of my most peaceful and relaxing moments come when I'm out in nature. Walking calms, releases stress, and helps fight anxiety and depression. However, the researchers found that those who practiced yoga had double the levels of GABA than the walkers.[33]

---

[31] GABA. (n.d.). Retrieved August 13, 2015, from http://www.denvernaturopathic.com/news/GABA.html

[32] Seligson, S. (2010, September 1). Your Brain on Yoga: Calmer, More Content | BU Today | Boston University. Retrieved August 13, 2015, from http://www.bu.edu/today/2010/your-brain-on-yoga-calm-er-more-content/

[33] Streeter, C., Whitfield, T., Owen, L., Rein, T., Karri, S., Yakh-kind, A., . . . Jensen, J. (n.d.). Effects of Yoga Versus Walking on Mood,

And as for yoga teachers and avid yogis, you're in luck; the study showed that those who were teachers and those who had practiced yoga for a long time were able to release GABA quicker than the newer practitioners.

Due to the deep breathing, the focusing, and the Yoga moves all combined together, you get a wonderful release of natural GABA. This calms your body's central nervous systems, keeps your stress levels low, and helps you get rid of stress quicker when your stress levels rise.

For those of you who have heard about GABA may also know that GABA is neurotransmitter that plays a key role in growth hormone (GH) secretion. GH is a powerful anabolic hormone that builds lean mass, melts body fat, and enhances athletic performance. Many people try supplementing with GABA but since it does not cross the blood brain barrier your money on supplements is wasted. As an athlete and person who is extremely interested in your health, making the most of your workouts and building a nice, strong, lean body, it would behoove you to take a couple of yoga classes each week, preferably one each day/evening.

There are GABA supplements sold at stores, but no evidence confirms that taking a GABA supplement can change your GABA levels. In fact, "Current medical opinion says that GABA taken as a supplement does not reach the brain and has no effect or benefit aside from being a benign placebo."[34] So *save* your money on the pills and head to a yoga class.

I named my studio Solace, which means peace, because yoga calms down the body. Since it gave me peace, I wanted to share that gift of

---

Anxiety, and Brain GABA Levels: A Randomized Controlled MRS Study. Retrieved August 13, 2015, from http://www.ncbi.nlm. nih. gov/pmc/articles/PMC3111147/

[34] GABA. (n.d.). Retrieved August 13, 2015, from http://www. denvernaturopathic.com/news/GABA.html

peace with others. I wish more people would turn to yoga rather than alcohol or food when they become stressed.

Once when I was at an amusement park, I saw a young girl wearing a shirt that said, "I do yoga to relieve stress. No, I'm just kidding, I drink wine." I wanted to trip her so that when she fell, she would have some sense knocked into her. No, I'm just kidding, that's not very yogic.

Old, young, fat, skinny, injured, athletic, everyone would greatly benefit from the practice of yoga. I encourage you to learn more about the philosophy and practice of yoga. In the meantime, go to a class and practice the asanas (the third part of the eight-fold path of yoga), it has the power to calm you down and relax you. Who doesn't need that?

Benefits of Yoga

The asanas (poses practiced) in a yoga class help to:

- Detoxify the lymph system

- Strengthen the bones of the body

- Improve flexibility

- Strengthen the immune system

- Support digestive health

- Prevent joint injury by keeping you limber and joints healthy

Yoga is life changing in many ways. People come to it at different levels of fitness and at certain times in their life. Over the years of owning a yoga studio, I've gotten to know many of my clients personally, and I've learned that people come to yoga for many different reasons. Some come for their health. Others come for stress relief when they're going through a tough time in life. Others are moms that get in tune with their body when they become pregnant. The reasons vary, but the yoga path helps everyone in their own unique way.

My favorite aspect of yoga is that it helps you to develop your self-awareness. When you are on your mat, you begin to notice everything about your body. You notice how you move and how you breathe – your lung capacity. You notice if you have an off day with your energy. Yoga brings you in tune with your body. You become much more aware of your nutrition and your digestion, your attitude, your skin, and your muscles – pretty much everything.

Yoga helps people of all ages increase their fitness level. Whether you are an avid fitness enthusiast or a beginner, yoga can help you. The body benefits greatly from moving the joints, stretching, and putting tension on the muscles, bones, and joints. The movements in combination with the deep breathing calm and replenish many systems of the body, including your circulatory system, your lymphatic system, and your digestive system.

With continued practice, you will experience improved flexibility, strength, and range of motion, and you will begin to have a fantastic posture. I remember at a cookout a friend saying, "Dang! Posture!" because I was sitting up straight while everyone else was slumped into their chair.

Yoga also is great for those who have high-stress lives or those who are depressed. Yoga draws your focus inward to the mind and body. As I said before, it calms your central nervous system, more specifically it helps to quiet the sympathetic nervous system, which is the body's fight or flight response. Once you start to practice, your parasympathetic nervous system begins to counterbalance the sympathetic nervous system, restoring your body to a state of calm. Yoga can and will help you bring more peace into your life.

In addition, yoga can help manage chronic conditions. It has been proven to help people with a variety of health challenges such as anxiety, back pain, depression, cancer recovery, asthma, high blood pressure, arthritis, multiple sclerosis, and even insomnia.

Many of my yoga students report improvements in their chronic health challenges. My mom became a yoga teacher in 2013 after she had retired from the insurance industry. When she first came to yoga, she was experiencing problems with her neck. Because of chronic pain and deterioration of her cervical vertebrae, it looked like she would have to have surgery. She was 63 years old when she began her yoga practice. The first year she came, she was about six months away from having neck surgery. She went back to the doctor about nine months later, and the doctor said, "Whatever you're doing, keep doing it because it's working. Come back and see me in a year." She was ecstatic because the yoga helped her avoid neck surgery altogether.

Some people come to yoga classes for fitness and to balance their workout regimen between running and lifting weights. Other people come to yoga because they are struggling with a loss. A family member might have passed away, or they might have been through a breakup. Still others come because they want a spiritual practice. They wish to go a bit deeper into the connection between their mind and body. Whatever the reason is that you begin doing yoga, you will soon find that it is much more than a physical practice. It is a practice that leads you to hear your internal voice of your spirit and becoming in tune with this, in my opinion, is where the magic of life begins to happen.

Ancient yogis knew all along that when we get into our body and out of our head, we get into a zone where our mind slows down. Then we are open to receiving and hearing this inner voice.

One time I was on my mat, an ex-boyfriend popped into my mind. I immediately felt compassion for him. I started crying because of the way had I treated him at the end of our relationship. I had fallen in love with someone else and when I realized that, I ended the relationship very quickly. The end was a shock to him at the time. Later he understood why we weren't good for each other, but in that moment, I received the letting-go and healing I needed to move on.

Yoga helps us to become self-aware. Every person I know has become "softer" because of their yoga practice. They live less steered by their ego and more steered by their spirit. Yoga helps us to see our behavior and live a more compassionate life.

Where to Get Started with Yoga

I'm often asked questions like "How many times per week should I practice?" "Should I do hot yoga?" "Should I do it at home?" There is a difference between doing yoga home alone and doing it with a group of people. At home, you're bound to be distracted. When you do yoga with others in a studio, the sounds of the deep breathing, the focusing on the body, and the overall ambiance of the room is calming, so I advise people to head to a yoga studio. Some gyms try to incorporate yoga into a small room in the corner and in my professional opinion, this kind of yoga sucks. When you can hear what is going on outside of the room those distractions keep you from experiencing the true benefits of going within.

As I said, yoga is a way of life, so I recommend people to practice yoga in some form every day. I teach my yoga school students that meditation should be a daily practice as well and that it is part of the path of yoga. I also recommend going to classes at least two to three times per week minimum. If you have a lot of stress in your life, then you should be going to a class every single day until your stress levels come down.

When you do yoga, it's important to go to a class that suits your level. If you are a beginner, you should go to a beginner's class so that you can get an understanding of the Sun Salutation Sequence and what the different poses are. When you know this sequence, you can feel better about attending any class, and from there you can determine what you need. Perhaps you want a gentle practice. Or if you want a proper workout, you can find intermediate to advanced level classes. They will indeed give you the butt kicking that you are looking for. In some yoga classes, such as yin or kundalini, you perform very few yoga poses. I like to tell clients that are new to my studio to give each class a try because they might find there are many classes they like.

It's important to go to a class that is taught by a certified yoga teacher. Teachers should be certified by the National Yoga Alliance. If they are certified by this alliance, you will see the letters E-RYT or RYT after their name. The certification means that they have had proper training in anatomy, physiology, the yoga path, and most of the yoga poses. In addition to the physical, certified yoga teachers will have been exposed to the philosophy of the ancient yoga tradition.

I recommend yoga to every person I meet because of its many benefits. To me, yoga is a way of life. The physical practice helps the body in many ways and leads to the focusing of the mind. Right now, I practice the yoga poses (called asanas) about five days per week on top of my figureFIT! workouts. Yoga is the No. 1 thing I would do if I could not lift weights anymore because you are lifting and moving your own body weight, which is just as good for you as lifting weights in the gym.

Once you're a member of the figureFIT! program, will have access to yoga videos in the yoga library. There you will find beginner videos that teach the Sun Salutation Sequence, and you will also find videos that show how to do more challenging poses such as chaturanga. You can work with these poses in the comfort of your home at any time of day that suits you best.

Yoga is a gift and many men shy away from it because they think it's a female practice and boy-oh-boy that is such an ego thing. Get over yourself gentlemen, you need yoga too. Here let me fluff your ego a little bit, yoga started with men. Yes indeed, it was spread all across the world via men. Yoga was initially brought to Chicago, LA & NYC and once all the rich female housewives in Hollywood latched on to it - it swept the nation. It's sad that people feel the need to segregate things out as feminine and masculine but they do. Well, I'll tell you what, smart men do yoga!

CHAPTER 15
How to Stay on Track

We're human. We see something we want, and we go full speed towards that goal. Sometimes we reach our goal and other times we get discouraged and give up. I see it time and time again with people who start fitness or nutrition programs. They start off great, and then they fizzle out.

What happens? Stress. Life. We are an overworked, over-stimulated, and underplayed society. We may have goals but when stress hits, we go back to old habits and easy choices. It's not just something weak people do; everyone does it. We all are victims of stress and the automatic mode of the brain.

The brain has been building procedures to help us our whole life. But sometimes those procedures are not serving us. This is where self-awareness comes into play. We must look at what unfolds when stress hits. What do we turn to? Do we turn to the couch? Shopping? What foods do we turn to? Chips? Sugar? Alcohol? Knowing what you do when stress hits is imperative to your breaking bad habits. To help you, I've created the worksheet "Breaking Bad Habits," which you will find in the back of the book. Self-awareness is key, and I use my stop, drop and meditate technique when I catch myself in the middle of doing something that I know does not serve me.

Deciding small behaviors that you are willing to do is also a key. You need to identify the process that you are willing to go through. If you're not willing to do one of my workouts to get you out of a funk, what are you willing to do? You need to find something that will help you bring your energy to a place that serves you and makes you feel good.

When you are in a place where you feel good, you are more willing to do the things that are in your best interest. You are more willing to get back on track. It's when you remain in a negative headspace that you will not move forward. You will fall off the wagon, and you will stay there unless you do something to get you back up. When you keep moving forward in the direction of your goals, even if you are crawling, you are still moving forward. Not every day or week is a good one. But the key is to forgive yourself quickly and align yourself with energy that will serve you and make you feel great.

You're not reading this book because you are comfortable with your life the way it is. You're reading it because something is calling you to change. Deep down you know there is a better way and you're looking to find it. The fact that you picked up this book, read it, and are now excited to change things about your life is proof that you must now put down some serious work to make your life and health the way you want it. Serious work, you ask? Yes, but it takes place in the daily process of life. Life is lived and enjoyed in the moment. So when you are not happy or enjoying life, I want you to go back to Chapter 2 and take a look at the things you wrote down that make you happy and the things you love and implement them daily.

Your life is your creation. The only way you will get the life you want is by doing the things that will give you the results you want.

It's easy to give up, but that's not the type of person you are. I know who you are, and that is why I wrote this book. You are a go-getter. You want more for your life, and you're willing to put in the work.

So how do we continue to succeed even when stress hits? *We plan! Then we implement the tools that make us happy every single day.*

Every day is a new day, and since this is a lifestyle, we must live it every day. We can't just put in 14 days, 33 days, or 165 days and say,

"Ok, I've put in my dues." No! We must do live this way every day. We must fill our physical, mental, and spiritual bank account every day so that we can be a person who gives back in all those areas. You will not and cannot serve when you are on empty. It's not possible.

I meet too many young women who are busy serving their families, husbands, and jobs, and they are miserable because they are not giving anything to their own self. It's not until those women get a bit older and perhaps go through a divorce (or two) that they *finally* decide to put themselves first. Know that you are not serving anyone when you are spiritually, mentally, and physically empty. You can be a great wife, mom, husband, dad, or partner when you take care of you. In fact, you will be a great partner because you will be happier.

In 2014, I had a big photo shoot for a magazine. Before the photo shoot, I was so rigid with my workouts and diet that once it was over, I went the other direction. I had no structure; I didn't have anything planned for about six months. Then I found myself floundering. I got lazy with my foods. I was eating whatever Paleo foods I wanted whenever I wanted to, and I wasn't keeping track of anything. My workouts were still happening, but they were not as focused as they were before. Then it hit me; I work very well under the pressure of a goal. Goals motivate me. Realizing this was key for me. I thought that I was doing well on this lifestyle program but realized that I was still living in the extremes.

This realization was a huge eye opener for me because the last thing I wanted was for my life to be extreme in any direction. I love balance and peace. I don't love killing myself to hit a goal. Fitness extremism or nutrition extremism must be banished. It has no place in the life of someone who chooses to be happy, healthy, and fit. I like to enjoy my life; otherwise what is the point? My whole goal in life is peace. I want peace more than anything. So when I find myself out of balance, it's time to find out why it happened and course correct.

After this incident, I dove into nutrient timing and got very clear about what to eat and when to eat it based on my workouts. I still ate the wonderful Paleo foods I was eating before. I simply timed the carbohydrates and fats more appropriately and once I knew this and started to live this way, my physique became effortless. I fine-tuned my workouts so that I was hitting every major muscle group. I also made sure that the figureFIT! workouts were created to strategically burn fat and keep me in that anaerobic zone, and building my metabolism. I continue to teach yoga a couple of times per week and practice at home as well nightly.

It's important to find your why behind all of this. You may be like me and needing to change your diet for your health, if so, do it and don't look back. You'll change the trajectory of your life and health. You may simply want to look great naked, awesome! There's no judgement, I totally get it and there's nothing wrong with wanting to look fantastic in a swimsuit. Models get paid for it, why can't we all? Maybe you just need more peace in your life… That will come as you begin to make new choices that serve your soul. Know this, in order for you to love your life, you must make deliberate choices about what you will do and when. Don't let life happen to you, create it.

My Tips & Tricks

I encourage you to do your best with following the figureFIT! meal guide in the back of the book. However, because everyone's needs are different, you may have to adjust portion sizes or move meals around to fit your schedule and activity level. If you feel unbearably hungry or experience low energy, don't be afraid to increase portion sizes or add a sixth meal.

Schedule your workouts as unbreakable appointments with yourself. Do not let anything other than a true emergency keep you from your workouts. Self-care is self-love and you can not serve the world when you never serve yourself.

Remove temptations – this is a must! Regardless of what your thing is: crackers, chips, sweets, wine or liquor you must take it out of the environment - this will eliminate the need for willpower. I tell my clients, if it's bad for you, it's bad for your kids too so don't buy it. When it is in the house, you know you'll find your way to it, so take the stimulus completely away - this will help you so much. If you can't get rid of the temptations, do your best to remove it from your sight. Designate a special cupboard to keep the foods you don't want to eat and then make it a no-go zone for you.

When you fail, because you will (we all do). Know that it is simply a place needing extra attention. As you shine the light on the weaknesses you can illuminate where they stem from. I like to sit in a meditation with the things that are bothering me. There, in the meditation, it is safe to feel the feelings, to get mad, to vent, to cry, and by doing so, you allow it to move through you. Once it moves through you, you grow past it.

Have a meal-prepping day. Prepping meals and having healthy and ready-to-eat foods on hand can stop you from making poor decisions. Prepping for the days ahead will help "set you up to win". Keep it simple by grilling chicken or your favorite fish, boiling eggs, and washing and chopping vegetables so that they're ready for you when you need them. On top of this, have your healthy meal replacement shakes on hand. I love when I'm busy and it takes me less than 5 mins to create my lunch - I can head right back to what I was working on and keep cranking out my work. If you would like to sign up for Isagenix, email us at info@figurefitlife.com to set up a time to get started with Isagenix (serious inquires only).

Keep track of your goals and foods in a fitness journal. I've created the "Daily Macronutrient Tracking Sheet," you can download this by visiting my website. I track my waters, meals, and vitamins everyday on one of these sheets. You may want to keep track of your life, emotions, and choices in a journal, not only to help you stay accountable in making a healthy lifestyle change, but also to help you discover what makes you feel your best. It goes WAY beyond writing down what you eat each day. In your journal, include the following:

a. How many hours of quality sleep you slept the night before - this will help you stay on track and avoid carb binges.

b. List what you're grateful for and watch as more comes to you.

c. Write down the #1 needle moving activity that you must get done that day for you.

d. What you ate and how it made you feel (great, bloated, etc)

e. What workout you will be doing that day

f. Keep a motivational quote in your sight to inspire you.

CHAPTER 16
The Tools: The Magic Is in the Doing

I believe that you began reading this book because you want to honor yourself and your body. You feel the need to change something or become more aligned with what you want out of this life. It's going to take daily effort on your part daily. Yes, *daily!* The magic is in the doing. You can wish all you want for things to change, but nothing will change until you put into action the tools that will propel you towards your highest goals and vision for yourself.

Progress means taking that first step. Mastery comes with consistency. No one person is a professional in their first attempt. I love the quote: "Entrepreneur: Someone who jumps off a cliff and builds a plane on the way down" (unknown).

Change happens only by taking action. But my motto is: "Baby steps to change." A champion puts in the work daily, not only when they want to. A champion builds this lifestyle into their life. Another phrase I tell my clients is "Happiness is our birthright." So be happy. Dance. Laugh. Eat healthy foods. Be kind. Work out *hard.* Engross yourself in the moment. Choose love over fear. Don't gossip – ever. Love people. Live life daily. Put the tools of happiness into place and then *live.* Don't wait to live or play because life is happening *now,* not when you reach your destination or goal.

It's when you commit to putting yourself first and love yourself that you will see drastic changes in your life and your body. The beauty is that it doesn't take a ton of time. When you do the *right* things, your body, life, and mind will fall into place and become exactly how you want them to be.

Only *you* can make the change. No one else does it for you. You must bring your dedication and will to change to this program and then follow the tools to create miraculous changes in your life. The *tools* are here in the figureFIT! Program: meditate, eat the right foods, train your body the right way, and connect to your tribe to give and receive support. When you put these tools into place and apply them consistently, you will begin to see your life through new eyes.

Consistency is key!

We are what we repeatedly do. Excellence, then, is not an act, but a habit. "
– Aristotle

The kind of lifestyle that you have read about in this book may take you well out of your comfort zone initially. But let me ask you something: Which discomfort would you prefer? Would you prefer taking steps out of your comfort zone and experience change, or would you prefer to continue telling yourself, "I hate the way I look; I can't fit into anything?" Which of these scenarios is the most uncomfortable for you?

I have reminders that go off on my phone every day that says, "Get uncomfortable!" It's my way of reminding myself daily that change does not happen when I am staying in my comfort zone. If I want to be a speaker at an event, I have to get over my fear, get uncomfortable, build the courage, and ask for what I want. When I have dared to take steps that felt uncomfortable, I have landed articles in magazines and received TV roles and speaking engagements (paid). It all happened because I put myself in a vulnerable position. Sometimes I was accepted. Sometimes the no's were not now's, but it has always led my life to a place of growth and dramatic change.

The *same* thing goes for the body. You can't change unless you are willing to be uncomfortable and sweat a little bit every day.

Sometimes getting uncomfortable is the workout I am not feeling up to. Sometimes it is conquering the fear of going bigger and trying something that I have always dreamed of trying. So let me ask you, where can you challenge yourself to get uncomfortable?

Are you ready to be accountable to yourself? Are you ready to show up and look at yourself in the mirror and say, "_____ *(insert your name), I love you. Your life is a gift. I am ready to take care of you and respect you every single day for the rest of my life."*

You're invited to join the rest of the figureFIT! tribe over at figureFITlife. com. We look forward to meeting you, hearing your story, and watching you evolve along with all the rest of us on this magical journey called life. We are here to support you, love you, and help you face your bad habits, break them, and create new life-affirming habits that are going to rock your world and help you to create the best life, mind, and body.

I can promise you that when you join the figureFIT! Lifestyle Program, you will change your life, and you will become happy, healthy, and FIT! The magic is in the doing; so come on over and sign up, I can't wait to support you.

Much love to you, my new friend!

Please come over and join me in a discussion on Facebook, Twitter, Instagram, LinkedIn, Periscope, and anywhere else you like to play on social media. I want to connect with you. Look for @liznierzwicki and @figurefitlife.

Join the figure*FIT!* 90-Day Transformation Challenge

I used to cry in my closet because I was "too fat" for my clothes. I killed calories in the gym after binging the night before. I've scolded myself time and time again over my body, but none of that ever worked.

It wasn't until I started seeking help from people who had the body, health, and life I wanted that my life began to change. I dove into books, seminars, and classes to help me learn how to better myself. I hired life, fitness, and nutrition coaches. Some were good, and some were great while others didn't seem to give me a second glance or care about my goals. Eventually, I started learning how to love myself through proper care such as positive thinking, eating the foods that were right for me (listening to my body's signals), and working out the right way.

After years on this journey, I realized I needed to create my own program to help clients because none of the one's I came across or that I signed up for helped with these major issues: digestive health, breaking bad habits, and proper workouts. I wanted to create a program that fully integrated fitness, digestive health, healing, and a healthy mindset - so I created exactly what I would have wanted help with when I was hiring my coaches. Now here it is *for you!*

With this book *and* my online program, you receive the tools you need to create a solid foundation for a happy mind, a healthy gut, and a strong, sexy body. When you head over to figurefitlife.com and join the online figureFIT! Lifestyle Program, you will receive all the tools you need to make major changes in your life. You will also have direct access to me on a daily basis via the private group page on Facebook.

Change does *not* happen in your comfort zone, so it's time to commit to you, your goals, and your health and start taking steps daily for your happiness and health.

Here is what you receive:

- Three figureFIT! Metabolic Conditioning Workouts per month

- Weightlifting Workouts

- A Monthly Fitness Calendar

- Yoga Videos

- Audio Meditations (self-awareness is key!)

- The figureFIT! Nutrition Guide with Food Lists

- Paleo Recipes

- Private group support page for daily check-ins and support

- Motivating Group Coaching Calls

Enter to Win:

To enter the challenge, simply head to figureFITlife.com and click on the 90-Day Transformation tab. I can't wait to support you on your journey.

APPENDIX

figure*FIT!*
Worksheet I

Acknowledge Your Limiting Beliefs

Understand where you are playing the victim. It's time to start noticing your excuses – the things that you tell yourself. Write down everything you think hinders you from moving forward. If you are unsuccessfully trying to lose weight, you might be telling yourself, A, I am on the pill. B, I travel too much. C, I have to take clients out for work. D, I do not have enough time. Another excuse could be, "I can't cook healthy food because my kids won't eat it," or "I'm big-boned, it runs in my family," or "I'm too tired after work to go to the gym." These are stories that people tell themselves. Now it is time to start telling a new story.

We are human, so having limiting beliefs is normal. This exercise is not an opportunity to pass judgment on yourself but an opportunity to grow.

1. Acknowledge stories that you tell yourself about why you can't have the body you want.

(Example: I do not have time.)

2. Write down a fear or limiting belief about yourself. (Example: "People don't like me," "I'm afraid of rejection," or "I'm afraid of what people think.)

_____

_____

_____

_____

3. Consider the following questions:

    - How has this belief held you back?

    _____

    _____

    _____

    - What has this cost you so far?

    _____

    _____

    _____

    - How has holding onto this story falsely served you (kept you in your comfort zone)?

    _____

    _____

    _____

    - How would you feel without this limiting belief?

    _____

    _____

    _____

    - What would you do (or accomplish) if you were free of this limiting belief?

    _____

    _____

    _____

Now it is time to shatter your limiting beliefs and break down those excuses.

For every limiting belief or excuse, come up with a *new* affirmation (thought) that you will tell yourself when this old story comes up. Make this affirmation in the present tense so that you can give it power and energy.

Examples:

Story: "I don't have time to work out."

Affirmation: "I have just as much time as everyone else – even the top fitness models. I create time for what is important to me."

Or

Fear: "I don't think people like me."

Affirmation: "I have many loving relationships and am loved."

Fear:_____

_____

_____

Affirmation:_____

_____

_____

Fear:_____

_____

_____

Affirmation:_____

_____

_____

figureFIT!
Worksheet II

Set Yourself Up to Win

Fill out one sheet per goal.

1. What is my most important goal?_____
   _____
   _____

2. What is my deepest desire to realize this goal? What is the big
   picture of my life and my *"why"*? _____
   _____
   _____

3. What specific actions am I willing to take to achieve this goal?
   (These are actions such as taking lunch every day to work, going to
   the gym right after work, and carrying a gallon of water around to
   drink more water. These are called behavioral commitments.) ____
   _____
   _____
   _____
   _____

4. When, where, and how am I willing to take these actions? _____
   _____
   _____
   _____
   _____

5. What is the biggest obstacle that can get in my way? What are other obstacles that could get in my way?_____

_____

_____

_____

_____

6. What will I do when this obstacle arises?_____

_____

_____

_____

_____

Now take the time to write down your goal and plan your commitments. Also plan your setbacks and how you will overcome them. Then visualize your goal and any obstacles. Visualize what you will do when those obstacles arise and how you will overcome them. *This is the most powerful step in achieving your goals.*

Prepare to Win (Examples)

What is likely to come up this week that can throw me off with my workouts?

Example: My son's basketball game may tempt me to eat the pizza that will be on hand.

Example: My meeting may run late causing me to miss my workout on Wednesday.

What will I do if this thing happens?

Example: I will eat before the game and put gum in my mouth at the game to remind myself that I do not want the pizza.

Example: I will walk for a minimum of 20 minutes that morning just in case my meeting runs over causing me to miss my workout. If I do miss the workout, I can make it up on Saturday morning when my schedule is free, and I will promise myself to get it done.

Creative Use of Reminders

You can set reminders on your calendar, iPhone, or any other device to help you stay on track.

Example: Since I tend to eat more at night. At 6:00 PM, I have set reminder in my phone to help me stick true to my goals of eating healthy. Here are some examples of what my reminders say:

"I eat healthy foods. My health is important to me." "A fit body is sexy."

"I build my meals around clean, healthy foods."

What are some reminders that resonate with you? Write them down. More importantly, put them somewhere you can see them!

1.

2.

3.

Engage Daily with Your Accountability Partners (figureFIT! Private Group Page on Facebook)

The figureFIT! Program comes with a tribe to help you succeed. We are like-minded individuals on a mission to health, happiness, and a FIT body.

Are you checking in on the private group page? Set reminders to post on the page daily.

figure*FIT!*
Worksheet III

Breaking Bad Habits

figureFIT!

Breaking Bad Habits

By Liz Nierzwicki

*Hi! My name is Liz Nierzwicki, founder of Solace Yoga Studio. Creator of figureFIT! and the author of the best-selling book, **Happy Healthy FIT Transform Your Life in 90-Days.** I want nothing more than to help you create a life that you love; a life that is filled with happiness and contentment; a life that allows you to enjoy the journey and chase your dreams knowing that you are completely supported by the Universe.*

*I'm currently writing my second book, **Bad Habit Breaker**, a book that teaches you how we initially created our bad habits (how they develop in the brain) and then how to BREAK THEM and create new habits. I couldn't wait to get you this worksheet, so here it is. Use this worksheet for the bad habits that are causing suffering in your life.*

You don't have to live with this struggle...

-Comfort eating   -Shopping Addiction
-Sex Addiction   -Drug Addiction
-Anger Issues   -Control Issues
-Procrastination   -Worry or Fear

3-Steps to Breaking Your Bad Habits

1.) Recognize The Process That Unfolds

Start by catching yourself in the process...
How does the process unravel?
What happened before you engaged in this habit?

2.) What Did the Impulse Feel Like?

What did the initial impulse (to engage in this bad habit) FEEL like?
Sit and think about the feelings that came up?
What sensations arose within your body?
What feeling are you trying to avoid?

3.) What Was the Trigger?

What was the initial trigger that made you turn to this habit?
When we know what triggers us to engage in the habit we are able to prevent OR choose to something else. Then . . .

figurefitlife.com   Mindset Coaching   gutHEALTH   Energy System Training

STOP DROP & MEDITATE

When you understand your triggers, you are then more likely to notice when a feeling or sensation arises within you to want to turn to this negative behavior. When you notice this trigger or impulse, deploy the *Self-Awareness Meditation* - this meditation can be found at figurefitlife.com under the meditation tab! *The key to change is building self-awareness through slowing down the process and watching how it all unfolds.*

Ask yourself the following questions and write down your answers:

1.) When did I last engage in this bad habit?

2.) What triggered my actions?
(This is not an opportunity to pass blame, we take full responsibility of our own actions here at figureFIT!)

3.) What did the initial impulse or sensation feel like?

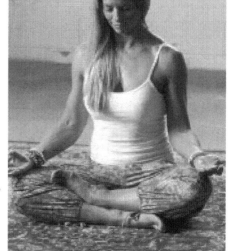

Photo by Paul Buceta

4.) What did you say to yourself about yourself or another person?

5.) How did the process unfold?
(what did you do)?

6.) What basic survival need is this trying to meet?
(Hunger, Fear, Love, Worth, Self-Defense, Sexual)

7.) How well is this behavior meeting this need?

8.) If you were free of this bad habit, what might you do instead?

5 Steps to Creating New Habits

1.) What is your big goal?
What are your reasons behind this goal?

2.) What is the process you are willing to live?
What are you willing to do? To change you must find things you are willing to do instead that are healthy and help you enjoy life.

3.) What Behavioral Commitment can you put into place to help you create a new habit?
This step is the most important when creating a new habit. The brain likes to help us build procedural memories to make our life easier. So when you set up behavioral commitments, your brain will go to work helping you stick to those commitments.

"I will do_____when_____."

Example: *"I will pack my gym bag and take it to work with me every day so that when I am on my way home, I will have everything I need to go to the gym." OR "I will take a salad with lean protein to work every single day." Or "I will not smoke in my car anymore."*

4.) Visualize Your Success
The brain does not know the difference between actually doing something and imagining it, so when you visualize yourself doing something, you literally tell the brain what is going to happen and the brain starts to build a procedure for that thing you will do.

5.) Imagine the Obstacle (most important step)
It is important to know what has the potential to throw you off. So take a moment to write down what is likely to get in the way of your goals and what you will do WHEN this comes up.

Example: *"I am likely to get derailed when my co-workers ask me to happy hour. So I will politely decline and ask them to join me in the gym instead." OR "I am likely to get derailed when I do not take my gym bag to work with me. So if this happens, I will make sure to have a snack 45 mins before I am supposed to leave, head home, change, then head to the gym immediately so that I do not get in my own way."*

All of the five steps listed will help the brain create new habits. A habit is formed by you doing something, enough times that the brain makes is an automatic process. A habit is also something that initially gave you some sort of comfort even if that thing isn't necessarily good for you. When you do the above steps you help the brain break a bad habit in its track and then build a new habit by committing to new behavioral commitments.

*The science behind how this works will be broken down in my book: **Bad Habit Breaker** (releasing in late 2015). Make sure you're signed up for my newsletter at figurefitlife. com so that you can get advanced notification as to when the book will be released. If you're interested in getting more help on your fitness or weight loss journey, join me here: figurefitlife.com and sign up for the monthly online figureFIT! Lifestyle Program; where you get ME as your coach! I give you workouts (videos that will show you how to do the moves), a nutrition manual, weight training routines, yoga videos, meditations to help your mind, and unlimited support. You can do these workouts at home or the gym. It's time to build your best body, develop a healthy focused mind, and create a happy life beyond your wildest dreams!*

figurefitlife.com   Mindset Coaching   gutHEALTH   Energy System Training

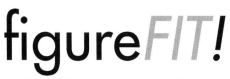

I Have the Power to Choose Me

Event Planning Sheet - Preparing for things that have the potential to throw me off

What throws you off?

_____

_____

What can you do before hand to prepare you for this occurrence?

_____

_____

What will you do instead when faced with this challenge?

_____

_____

What will I say if I'm questioned? Or what will I say to myself?

_____

_____

How will I feel when I make the right choice for me?

_____

_____

What will I remember about my life, my goals, or myself when this happens?

_____

_____

- Know your common derailments.
- Make a list of every question, concern, or objection that other people could possibly come up with to derail you.
- Remember projection is real - if your choice is a "no," - then you don't owe anyone an explanation. Period.
- Make a list of everything that could go wrong.
- Develop positive responses to all the negatives you've thought of.
- Have your plan (this sheet of paper) - take it out if you need a mental reminder. You never know- you may help someone else too when they see you following the plan.
- Take great confidence that you will succeed.

Tonight when you lay your head on your pillow, say this to yourself:

"Thank you (   ), you did a fantastic job today. I am proud of you."

figureFIT! Paleo Food Guide

Notes: CP: Cold Pressed   *: FODMAPs   *Italics: Fightshade Foods*

Meat, Seafood & Eggs

Beef	Ostrich	Clams	Shrimp
Bison	Pork	Grouper	Snapper
Boar	Quail	Halibut	Swordfish
Chicken	Rabbit	Lobster	Tuna
Duck	Squab	Mackerel	Limit:
Eggs	Turkey	Mahi Mahi	Bacon/Sausage
Wild Game	Veal	Mussels	Limit:
Goat	Venison	Oysters	Deli Meats/Jerky
Goose	Catfish	Salmon	
Lamb	Carp	Sardines	
Mutton	Cod	Scallops	

Fruits

Apples*	Grapefruit	Orange	Raspberries
Apricots*	Grapes	Papaya	Star Fruit
Avocados*	Kiwi	Passion	Strawberries
Bananas	Lemon	Peach*	Tangerine
Blackberries*	Lime	Pears*	Watermelon*
Blueberries	Lychee*	Pineapple	Limit: Dried Fruit
Cherries	Mango*	Plantain	
Cranberries	Melon (All Varieties)	Plum*	
Figs	Nectarine*	Pomegranate	

Vegetables

Artichokes*	Celery	Kale	Rutabaga
Asparagus*	Chard	Leeks*	Seaweed
Arugula	Collard greens	Letuce(red, etc.)	Shallots*
Bamboo shoots	Cucumbers	Lotus roots	Snap peas
Beets	Dandelion Greens*	Mushrooms*	Spinach
Bok choy	*Eggplant*	Mustard Greens*	Squash
Broccoli*	Endive	Okra*	Sugar snaps
Brussel sprouts*	Fennel*	Onions*	Sweet potatoes
Cabbage*	Garlic	Parsley	Tomatoes
Carrots	Green beans	Parsnips	Turnips
Cassava	Green onions*	*Peppers*	Watercress
Cauliflower*	Jicama*	Radicchio	Zucchini

Nuts & Seeds

Almonds	Flax seeds	Pine Nuts	Sunflower Seeds
Brazil nuts	Hazelnuts	Pistachios	Walnuts
Cashews	Macadamia nuts	Pumpkin Seeds	Any Listed = Nut Butter
Chestnuts	Pecan	Sesame Seeds	

Liquids

Water	Mineral Water	Almond Milk
Herbal Teas	Coconut Milk/Water	Organic Coffee

Herbs & Spices

Allspice	Chives	Horseradish/	Paprika
Anise	Cilantro	Wasabi	Pepper
Basil	Cinnamon	Juniper Berry	Peppermint
Bay Leaf	Clove	Lavender	Spearmint
Caraway	Coriander	Lemongrass	Rosemary
Cardamom	Cumin	Lemon Verbana	Sage
Carob	Curry	Licorice	Tarragon
Cayenne Pepper	Dill	Mace	Thyme
Celery Seeds	Fennel	Marjoram	Turmeric
Chervil	Fenugreek	Mint	Vanilla
Chicory	Galangal	Mustard	Vinegar
Chili Pepper	Garlic	Nutmeg	
Chipotle Powder	Ginger	Oregano	

Superfoods

Grass-Fed Dairy:	Sea Vegetables:	Bone Broth:	Fermented Foods:
Butter	Kelp	Homemade	Sauerkraut
Ghee	Seaweed	(not in can or box)	Carrots
	Herbs		Beets
Organ Meats:	Spices		High-Quality Yogurt
Liver			Kefir
Kidneys			Kombucha
Heart			

Fats & Oils

Avocado oil	Coconut Milk	Ghee	Flax Oil
Bacon Fat/Lard	Coconut Oil	Macadamia Oil	Sesame Oil-CP
Butter	Duck Fat	Olive Oil-CP	Walnut Oil

Sweets

Carob powder	Raw honey	Molasses
Cocoa powder	Maple syrup	Dark Chocolate

Food Preparation Tips

After the grocery: take an extra 30-60 mins to prepare your vegetables and fruits. Clean them, cut them into servings, and get them ready to be used when you need them.

For easy lunches: make a huge salad and store the salad in a large sealable container. Each morning prepare a single serving from the large batch and then mix in 1 serving of meat (Ex: beef slices, chicken, bison, salmon, tuna) Toss with a little olive oil and lemon juice and you are set.

Desserts: Berries and other fruits make a great dessert. Get creative. Pre-cut carrot and celery sticks, sliced fruit, and pre-portioned raw nut/dried fruit mixes are easy snacks.

Sample Meal Examples

Start your day with a 16oz of warm water. Warm lemon water, or a calcium/magnesium drink.

Breakfast: Start your day with a 16oz of water. Make an easy omelet. Sauté onion, peppers, mushrooms, and broccoli in olive oil; add free-range eggs (or egg whites and 1 yolk).

Snack: Sliced lean beef, vegetables or 1/2 serving of seasonal fruit and water.

Lunch: Large salad loaded with vegetables and 1 serving of lean meat or fish (olive oil and lemon dressing), herbal tea, or water. You can always use leftover dinner from the night prior for lunch.

Snack: Apple slices, raw walnuts.

Dinner: Tomato and avocado slices; grilled chicken breast; steamed broccoli or asparagus, carrots, and artichokes.

DAILY TARGET FOOD GUIDE

BEST FOODS • Incorporate into most meals, every day

Carbohydrates
Steel-Cut Oats
Quinoa
Whole Grain Rice
Spirulina
Spinach
Lentils
Sprouts
Chlorella
Yams/Sweet Potatoes
Flax Meal
Millet
Amaranth

Fruits
Berries
(Black/Blue/Raspberries)
Kiwi/Prunes

Vegetables
Most Vegetables
Spinach
Broccoli
Sea Vegetables

Protein
Wild Caught Fish
Wild Game
Organic Free-Range Eggs
Walnuts/Almonds
Pumpkin Seeds

Fats
Extra Virgin Olive Oil
Evening Primrose Oil
Extra Virgin Coconut Oil
Cod Liver Oil
Olives
Fish Oil
Avocado

Others
Garlic
Ginger

BETTER FOODS • Choose These Daily

Carbohydrates
100% Whole Wheat
Whole Grains
Kashi Buckwheat
Root Vegetables
Redskin Potatoes
Legumes
Beans

Fruits
Cranberry
Peach
Lemon/Lime
Orange
Grape Fruit
Mango
Green Apple
Watermelon
Pear
Grapes
Melon

Vegetables
Celery
Onion
Tomato
Carrots
Cucumber

Protein
Organically Raised
Cold Water Fish
Rice/Goat Protein
Organic Poultry
Tofu
Buffalo
Pine Nuts
Brazilian Nuts
Hazelnuts
Most nuts and seeds
Organic Goat Cheese

Dairy
Organic Milk
(Rice, Almond, Goat, Oat)
Organic Yogurt (Plain)
Greek Yogurt (Plain)

Fats
Almond Butter
(All Natural)
Macadamia Nut Oil
Flaxseed Oil
Sunflower Oil

Others
Green Leaf Stevia

GOOD FOODS

Carbohydrates
Quick Oats
Whole Grain Cereal
(<10g sugar/serving)
Corn (non GMO only)

Fruits
Raisins
Natural Applesauce
Fruit Spreads
Bananas
Red Apples

Vegetables
String Beans

Protein
Nitrate Free Deli Meat
Organic Lean Red Meat
(sirloin, round, flank)
Free-Range Eggs
Soy/Whey Protein
Powder (non GMO only)
Crab/Lobster
Farm Raised Fish
Peanuts

Dairy
Organic Dairy
Cottage Cheese

Fats
Natural Peanut Butter
Expeller Pressed Canola Oils
(non GMO only)
High Oleic Sunflower and Saf-
flower Oil
Organic Butter
Canola/Soy Mayonnaise

Others
Red Wine
Molasses
Organic Honey
Pickles
Dark Chocolate
(80% or higher)

FAIR FOODS • Choose Occasionally (Less Than 2X/Week)

Carbohydrates	Protein	Fats
White Potatoes	Canadian Bacon	Egg Yolk
English Muffins	Poultry Sausage	Cream Cheese
White Bread, Rice or Pasta	Pork Tenderloin	Butter
Rice Cakes	Nitrate Free Ham or Bacon	Mayonnaise
Pretzels	Organic Hot Dogs	Corn Oil
Mac & Cheese	Lean Ground Meat	Soybean Oil
Refined Granola Bars	Poultry	Cottonseed Oil
Pizza	Soy Nuggets	
	Eggs	**Others**
Fruits	Shrimp	White Wine
Apple Juice		Organic Sugar
Orange Juice	**Dairy**	
Grapefruit Juice	Whole Dairy Products	
	Processed Cheese	
Vegetables	Low Fat Dairy Products	
Iceberg Lettuce		

POOR FOODS • Eliminate from Diet or Have ONLY Occasionally

Carbohydrates	Protein	Fats
Potato Chips	Pork Sausage/Ham	Fried Food
Microwave Popcorn	Fatty Cuts of meat	Processed Cheese
Crackers	Fast Food Burgers	Hydrogenated Oils
Croissants/Pastries	Hot Dogs	Refined Peanut Butter
Baked Goods/Cakes		Non Dairy Creamers
Cookies	**Sugary Drinks/Sweets**	Margarine
Doughnuts	Milk Chocolate	Shortening
Sugared Corals	Soft Drinks	Gravy
Canned Fruits in Syrup	Diet Soda	Fat Free Ranch Dressing
	Candy	Fast Food Burgers/Fries
	Artificial Sweeteners	
	White Sugar	
	Ice Cream	

Meal Guide for Busy People

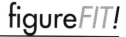

Please Note: The following meal guides are only suggestions. Keep starches before and after workout. The important part is that you keep the meal's food pairings the same and have no fat immediately after your workout.

Option 1

Meal 1:	Meal 2:	Meal 3:	Meal 4:	Meal 5:
Protein Fat Veggies 16oz glass of water, green tea or lemon water	Protein Good Fat Veggie or Fruit 16oz glass of water, green tea or lemon water	Protein Starch 16oz glass of water, green tea or lemon water	Protein Veggie or Fruit Starch 16oz glass of water, green tea or lemon water	Protein Veggie Good Fat 16oz glass of water, green tea or lemon water

If your goal is weight loss-you will want to drop the starch from that last meal and limit your intake of fruits to before or after your workouts.

Option 2 - Keep it simple with Isagenix meal replacements

Meal 1:	Meal 2:	Meal 3:	Meal 4:	Meal 5:
Isagenix AM Ageless Essentials Vitamin Pack Isagenix Isalean (or IsaPRo)Shake (w/ Isa Greens, if desired) 16oz glass of water, green tea or lemon water	Protein Good Fat Fruit or Veggie 16oz glass of water, green tea or lemon water	Isagenix Isalean Shake (women) IsaLeanPro (men) 16oz glass of water, green tea or lemon water	Protein Veggie or Fruit OR Isagenix Isalean Shake or Bar 16oz glass of water, green tea, or lemon water	Protein Veggie Starch Good fat Isagenix PM Ageless Essentials Vitamin Pack 16oz glass of water, green tea or lemon water

Optional Isagenix Supplements

Pre-Workout or Morning Pick-Me-Up	**Isagenix Want More Energy** (before workout or as an afternoon pick-me-up) OR Isagenix E+Shot
Afternoon	Isagenix Ionix Supreme (Drink hot or cold once per day, either before your workout or anytime throughout the day when you need a pick-me-up!)
Night-Time	**Night-Time Belly Buster Snack*** 8oz Almond Milk and 1 scoop Isagenix IsaPro Shake or blend with ice (if desired) The combination of calcium and protein before bed is a great belly-fat blasting protocol. *This does not add extra calories to your day's total. While this can be used as a 6th meal, it should NOT replace any of your others.

www.figurefitlife.com

I highly recommend the Isagenix Athlete's Pak to give you the fuel and treats you need WHEN you need them. I also add the IsaDelights Dark Chocolate for when I need that sweet treat. To view products head over to **www.liznierzwicki.isagenix.com**

figure*FIT!*
Lifestyle Habits

I often talk to my clients about my non-negotiables. These are the things I put into play every day. I do not work out or eat healthy only when I want to; I do it consistently, and that is the biggest factor in success. This is a lifestyle program, not an "I'll do it when I want program." Yes, I talk about transforming your life in 90 days, but that is only the beginning. You must create a new sustainable life that will help you create and maintain the life, body, and health you want.

Use this worksheet to help you create *your* non-negotiables.

Beginner's Weekly Workout Schedule (Example):

Monday: figureFIT! Workout 1

Tuesday: yoga

Wednesday: figureFIT! Workout 2

Thursday: walk for one hour with the family

Friday: figureFIT! Workout 3

Saturday: AM jog or yoga

Sunday: walk for one hour with the family

Intermediate/Advanced Weekly Workout Schedule (Example):

Monday: figureFIT! Workout 1 and yoga

Tuesday: Weight Lifting: Leg Day 1 and abs

Wednesday: figureFIT! Workout 2

Thursday: chest, triceps, abs, and HIIT

Friday: figureFIT! Workout 3

Saturday: back, biceps, and yoga

Sunday: Leg Day 2

figure*FIT!*
Affirmations

I love the little things that help me to stay motivated and keep me on track. Use the remaining worksheets as extra tools to help you on your journey.

On each of the figureFIT! workouts, I have an affirmation that I like to say when I'm in the middle of the workout. It's easy to tell yourself, "This is hard." When you do so, your body believes it, and your energy declines. When I'm working out, I like to tell myself positive things such as, "I am creating my best body one minute at a time." This small shift in mental words creates a dramatic shift in your energy.

Here are some other affirmations that you can use to help you achieve your goals and create the best life possible through the positive power of affirmations.

"I enjoy being healthy and doing what is good for me."

Use this affirmation when you feel reluctant to do what you know is in your best interest. The desire to sabotage our efforts to improve ourselves comes from our resistance to change. Self-improvement brings new activities, friends, and other manifestations of change that we often resist when we fear the unknown. But on the other side of change is your goals achieved. Repeat this affirmation over and over until you believe it.

"I love and accept myself as a unique individual."

Use this affirmation when you feel that people are not accepting you, especially if it's because you are different from other people or because you want to be different. You do not need the acceptance of other people to love yourself. You can't change anyone else, so focus on being the good person that you are.

"My willpower is stronger than my bad habits."

Use this affirmation when you are struggling with long-held beliefs, habits, and compulsions. Our bad habits have been acquired over the years because (we thought) at one point they helped us cope with something. Use this affirmation to help you create new habits that support you in your efforts to happiness and health.

"I have the power to transform my life."

Use this affirmation when you notice resistance, either in yourself or others, to the idea of being able to change your life. Profound change usually comes in small increments over time. I often tell my clients "baby-steps every day is how you change your life." Keep a positive attitude as you repeat this affirmation, and you will be able to undo years of negative self-talk in record time.

"I accomplish anything I put my mind to and work towards."

Use this affirmation when you doubt yourself, your intelligence, your memory, or your ability to achieve your goals. Your situation is largely the result of how well you blend your logical and intuitive faculties to direct your actions. Add this action to this affirmation: Several times per day, concentrate on a mental image of something you would like to see coming into your life.

"I believe in myself now, always, and in all ways."

Use this when you feel like you have failed or when others seem to doubt your abilities. Your strengths and weaknesses are yours to experience and learn from in your own time. Accept yourself just as you are now, knowing that the mistakes you have made helped guide the direction of your personal growth.

"I let go of things that are no longer useful."

Use this affirmation when you are resisting letting go of outmoded ways of thinking and acting, and people who are taking advantage of your time, body, energy, and other resources. If you want new people, places, things, situations, and ideas to come to you, you must make room for them in your life. Until then, enjoy your newfound freedom and know that exciting things await you.

"I use criticism only to make things better."

Use this affirmation when you realize you are being critical or are the recipient of another's criticism. It's important to understand where we are in life; we can't improve unless we are able to see what needs improvement. However, when we forget to turn off our critical voice, we become someone who is sad and not fun to be around.

"I take my time to rest, relax, and rejuvenate."

Use this affirmation when you find that you are hurried, under pressure, overworked, or have not taken time for yourself. No matter what your situation or work is, you will be better balanced when you are well rested, fit, healthy, and take time do it correctly. Do not let exhaustion and self-reliance turn unto an illness, injury, or accident. Take the time to love you.

figure*FIT!*
Meditation for Releasing Fear

Once you identify your fears or limiting beliefs and have recognized how they hold you back, take the time to sit with each one in meditation or contemplation. See if you can notice where feelings arise within your body as you think about each fear. I have felt feelings arise in my belly, my left hand, and my chest.

Take a moment to breathe into the feeling for 60 seconds. Close your eyes and move into the feeling. As you feel the feeling for a minimum of 60 seconds, you may find that it goes away. Other times, the feelings may be intense, but you shouldn't run away from them. Feeling the feelings can help you to release their strong hold on you. The ego loves to keep us stuck, small, and thinking we cannot change. But the spirit within knows your potential and knows your worth. As you feel the fear and get comfortable sitting in it, you will begin to release it.

As you go through this process, it's important not to judge yourself or your fear. Instead, be the compassionate witness of your fear as you sit in a one to five-minute long meditation.

Start your meditation by saying,

"Holy Spirit, I surrender this fear (or limiting belief to you). I choose to see things differently and am open to seeing through your lens."

Sit and breathe. Repeat this phrase throughout your meditation.

You may notice that you gain clarity around this feeling as you move into it. And you may find that as you do this meditation, the feelings peak and then subside into a peaceful feeling where you know you're supported. The more you practice this meditation, the faster you will heal from the fears that hold you back. As you release the fear, it gives you freedom to open up into love and the fullness of who you are.

Made in the USA
Charleston, SC
18 March 2016